Surviving a Virus Plague

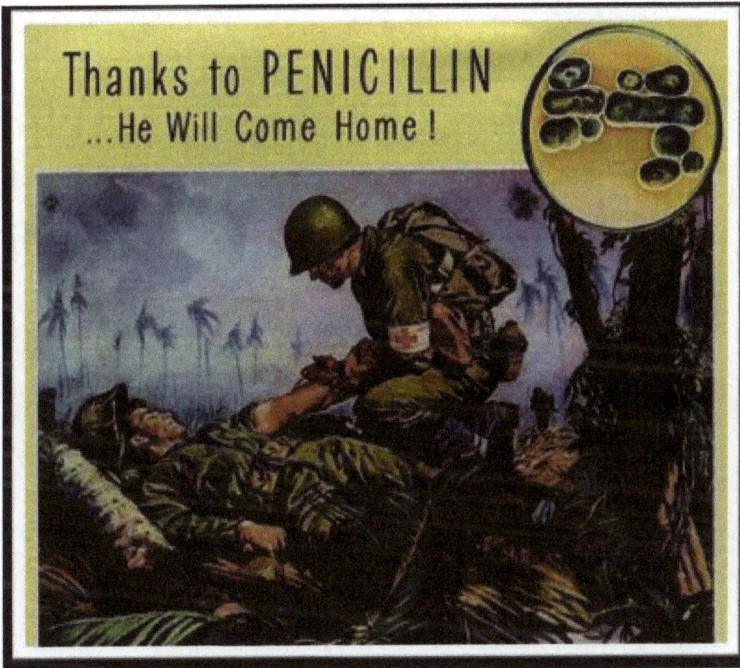

Thanks to PENICILLIN
...He Will Come Home!

The World War Museum

Copyright

Reference Study Guide

Contents

- Introudction ... **5**
- Virus symptoms: 10 key indicators and what to do ... **25**
- How to test for loss of smell? ... **34**
- How to make Penicillin ... **37**
- Foods that Fights Respiratory and Fungal Infections ... **67**
- Making Yogurt at Home for people with Diabetes ... **87**
- Virus Pandemics ... **97**
- How to make Insulin for Diabetes ... **105**
- Basic Principles of Ventilator Design ... **147**
- Position Virus/Lung Patients on their Stomach can save their Life ... 161

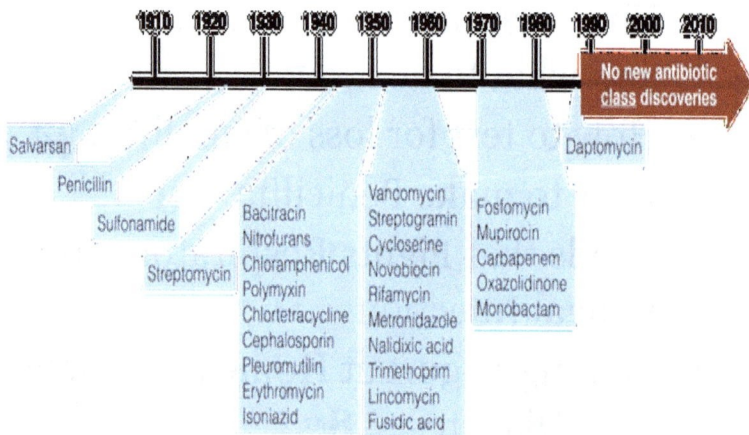

| | 1910 | 1920 | 1930 | 1940 | 1950 | 1960 | 1970 | 1980 | 1990 | 2000 | 2010 |

No new antibiotic class discoveries

Salvarsan

Penicillin

Sulfonamide

Streptomycin

Bacitracin
Nitrofurans
Chloramphenicol
Polymyxin
Chlortetracycline
Cephalosporin
Pleuromutilin
Erythromycin
Isoniazid

Vancomycin
Streptogramin
Cycloserine
Novobiocin
Rifamycin
Metronidazole
Nalidixic acid
Trimethoprim
Lincomycin
Fusidic acid

Fosfomycin
Mupirocin
Carbapenem
Oxazolidinone
Monobactam

Daptomycin

4

Introduction

We learned through the paranoia of our parents and teachers that disaster and doom were just around the corner in the form of giant earthquakes or a nuclear holocaust. We trained in school to crawl under our desks, as though this move would save us while everyone else was being vaporized by the blast. Many people bought into the bomb shelter idea. China and communism were always the greatest evil and surely will bring the world to a horrible end one day.

People that experienced the Great Depression knew the value of preparing for the worst. After the Great Depression people maintained a two-year stockpile of food and essential supplies, but later generations stopped doing that.

What constitutes a disaster is relative to the event and the effect it has on the individual or group. We, as Westerners in the Northern Hemisphere, are spoiled and prosperous. Even our poorest would be considered prosperous in the eyes of poorer people like in Gaza, Palestine. Our prosperous lives and governments shield us from discomfort and discontinuity. A drought in California just raises prices in America. A drought in Africa could kill millions. A disaster in Bangladesh would be an earthquake that crushes their huts, kills their children, and wipes out their village. A broken fingernail could be a disaster to a New England debutant.

A disaster is commonly defined as an event causing widespread destruction and distress. A grave misfortune. A crises event that surpasses the ability of an individual, community, or society to control or recover from its consequences.

For most North Americans a disaster is something nasty that happens to somebody else.

For those who need some coaching on the nature of disasters, here are some searing truths: (Bird Flu, Ebola, HIV, Swine Flu, Tsunamis, Hurricanes, Tornados) have reminded us, even in our protected cocoons of technological sophistication and prosperity, that we are virtually powerless in the face of nature and the entire region of the country can go from normality to catastrophe in the blink of an eye. Major disasters are a recurring fact of life for every generation, and the fact that we have not been visited by major disasters in the United States for two centuries only means that we are long overdue.

The fact is that we are not much more prepared in a practical sense to survive a long-term widespread disaster than our poorer counterparts in other counties who deal with similar situations on a daily basis.

Do you know how to survive?

- Do you have a survival cache of weapons and ammo? Your bug out bag is ready to go.
-
- Do you have food and water?

But will your demise be a simple cut or sinus infection?

Do you know how to make Antibiotics? Everything is OK until it is not OK. Then, it is a matter of how prepared you are to make things OK.

It was only a simple Scratch, but that is all it takes.

A little scratch on your hand can become a swollen, mess of pus after a few days of military-style sleep deprivation and poor hygiene. Within a day, a reddish purple line might appear from the pink scratch up to your forearm. Then a few hours later, the angry reddish line might reach your armpit. Then you might feel that you have a hangover from hell even though you had not drank in over a week.

Antibiotics changed life and medicine as we know it. Before Alexander Fleming's 1928 discovery of penicillin, there were a few options for the treatment of bacterial infections. Before Penicillin they cut off the limb or cut out that infected pound of flesh.

You could wait to see if your immune system wakes-up and destroys the germs. The body often does a pretty good job of defeating a lot of bugs.

However, your often body depends on everything being in good working order. A healthy immune system is well-fed, and well-rested. Diarrhea, a runny nose, fever, vomiting. These are all part of the body's attempt to destroy the germ, and to flush it out. But each of those things taxes your body heavily.

They use more of those valuable resources: Food, water, energy.

That is the guy in the zombie movie that everyone talks about leaving behind because he is slowing everyone down, and he probably will not make it anyhow.

Development of antibiotics for medical use began in the 1940's, and many illnesses moved from having a prognosis of certain death to a prognosis of 10 days of pill-popping as life goes on.

Prior to the 1940's your warning reddish line? Not good. So Which Infections Are Most Concerning? Even today, the death rate for septicemia is over 50%.

Bacterial skin infections (mostly staph infections) had a mortality rate of 10%. After the introduction of antibiotics, that death rate fell by 100 fold. How about Meningitis without antibiotics? Write your epitaph very quickly, before your brain gets cooked. However, to say that any bacterial infection untreated by Penicillin or antibiotics is a death sentence would be an exaggeration.

Other changes that seem so common sense to us now were just becoming the norm in the early 20th century like face masks, handwashing, at least times a day, house and room cleaning, proper garbage removal, sewage treatment, clean air, clean water, and vaccinations.

What do you think will disappear in our SHTF scenario?

- Will the garbage men still do their job?

- Will you be able to take that daily shower when life-giving water is scarce?

- When the grid goes down, will your home still be a comfy 78 degrees?

- Will you get your five servings of vegetables a day?

You get the point...things will be very bad.

A SHTF world is a pre-antibiotic world.

All of the things that helped improve the average lifespan from mid-forties in the early 20th century to nearly eighty in the early 21st century, sanitation, a steady food supply, a good night's sleep; they will be a thing of the past. But one big difference is that we can make Penicillin.

The question is: Will you have access to Penicillin or will you know how to make some? If you think ahead, if you prepare for the problem before you have the problem, you will be fine.

A Quick Antibiotic Lesson

There are two basic types of antibiotics: Broad-spectrum antibiotics and Narrow spectrum antibiotics. Think of it as a frag grenade versus a well-placed sniper shot.

- Broad-spectrum antibiotics kill most types of bacteria.

Doctors use these antibiotics when they cannot name that dog. If they do not know what kind of bacteria they need to kill, broad-spectrum antibiotics kill them all and let God sort them out. Broad-spectrum antibiotics are a good plan for those people who come into the ER so sick that antibiotics need to be getting to work within minutes and hours.

It is also a good plan for a layperson who knows that he or she has a bad bacteria but has no clue which bug is trying to kill him or her. The drawback with these is that your body plays the part of God and has to sort them out. Your body has to deal with a system that does not have good, bad, or ugly bacteria in or on it anymore.

Good bacteria does the following:

- It helps the skin stay healthy and keep the bad stuff out.
- Live in your gut and break down food so that you can absorb those nutrients.
- Act as an antibiotic of sorts by competing with and crowding out harmful bacteria.

The body has a lot of bacteria that are necessary for you to survive. Broad-spectrum antibiotics kill the good guys and the bad guys.

What can result from wiping out all your bacteria?

- Vaginal yeast infections. Good luck getting cranberry juice and yogurt in the SHTF world.

- Thrush. That's a yeast infection in your mouth. Yuck.

- Clostridium difficile "C-diff" an opportunist bacteria that grows when the good stuff disappears and causes terrible diarrhea. It kills 29,000 people every year.

All that besides the normal side effects that antibiotics have, like diarrhea (which actually evens out the constipation of a straight MRE diet), rash, and nausea.

Narrow spectrum antibiotics kill certain bacteria. In cases where the doctor is confident which bacteria needs treatment, these are the smart choice.

Narrow spectrum antibiotics will spare your good bacteria and keep you in the fight.

What are examples of narrow spectrum antibiotics? Examples of narrow-spectrum antibiotics are the older penicillins (penG), the macrolides and vancomycin.

Examples of broad-spectrum antibiotics are the aminoglycosides, the 2nd and 3rd generation cephalosporins, quinolones, and **synthetic** penicillins.

Azithromycin, for example, is a go-to for sinus infections. Did you know that some of your sinuses are separated from your brain by mere millimeters of bone tissue?

Doses of medications vary by person and by disease treated. For example, amoxicillin for a throat infection might be 250mg three times a day for seven days.

For a dental abscess, 500mg three times a day for five days. However, if you have kids, know that the doses will change as they grow.

WARNING! Antibiotic Resistance Is a Huge Problem

Superbugs are on the prowl and could lead us to a SHTF world. Antibiotic resistance is a huge problem and is more likely to destroy life as we know it than nuclear annihilation. Inappropriate use of antibiotics is a big problem. Doctors prescribe them for viruses because patients do not want to hear, "It's a virus. Drink fluids and rest."

Patients take seven days of antibiotics instead of the prescribed ten days because they feel better. What happens then? All that's left at the end of seven days are the bacteria that were able to resist the seven-day onslaught. The tough ones. The superbugs.

Plus, those germs recover and reproduce. Now we have MRSA, VRSA. Acronyms for bacteria so tough to kill that killing them may kill you in the process.

Bottom Line: Do not use your pet antibiotics to turn yourself into your own doctor!

Recognizing that a red line going up your arm as a bacterial infection does not put the M.D. behind your name.

Go to the doctor!

Also do some additional research. Know your medications and their limitations.

For example, most medications you can double the expiration date. If it expires in two years, it is probably good for four. It is best to store in the refrigerator.

Tetracycline, for example, becomes toxic to your kidneys after it has expired.

Before the SHTF, while we still live in a world that people are going to school for eight years to learn this stuff, you should not play doctor with your or your family's health just because you read an article on the internet. If you take antibiotics wrong, you might be the one that creates the Superbug.

Do not be Patient Zero!

Do not Be the One That Makes the Shit Hit the Fan.

However, after SHTF when doctors and medical supplies are rare (or non-existent) you better have a stash of survival antibiotics lying around for that sinus infection...just in case.

Plus, antibiotics will make an excellent survival bartering item. Just imagine how much your neighbor with a severe infection will trade you for a few fish antibiotics.

Virus symptoms: 10 key indicators and what to do

Fever, cough and shortness of breath are found in the vast majority of all Virus cases. Any or all symptoms can appear anywhere from two to 14 days after exposure to a virus.

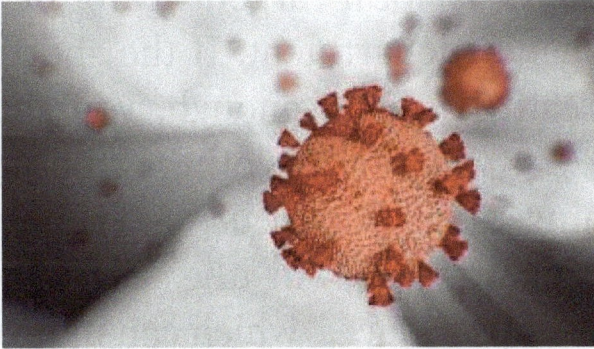

Here are 10 signs that you or a loved one may have a virus -- and what to do to protect yourself and your family.

1. Shortness of breath

Shortness of breath is not usually an early symptom of a virus, but it is the most serious. It can occur on its own, without a cough. If your chest becomes tight or you begin to feel as if you cannot breathe deeply enough to fill your lungs with air, that's a sign to act quickly, experts say. If there's any shortness of breath immediately call your health care provider, a local urgent care or the emergency department. If the shortness of breath is severe enough, you should call 911. There are other emergency warning signs for virus: a "persistent pain or pressure in the chest," and "bluish lips or face," which can indicate a lack of oxygen. Get medical attention immediately.

2. Fever

Fever is a key sign of a virus. Because some people can have a core body temperature lower or higher than the typical 98.6 degrees Fahrenheit (37 degrees Celsius), so do not to fixate on an exact number.

Most children and adults, however, will not be considered feverish until their temperature reaches 100 degrees Fahrenheit (37.7 degrees Celsius).

There are many misconceptions about fever. We all actually go up and down quite a bit during the day as much as half of a degree or a degree. Most people 99.0 degrees or 99.5 degrees Fahrenheit is not a fever.

Do not rely on a temperature taken in the morning. Instead, take your temperature in the late afternoon and early evening.

Our temperature is not the same during the day. If you take it at eight o'clock in the morning, it may be normal.

One of the most common presentations of fever is that your temperature goes up in the late afternoon and early evening. It is a common way that viruses produce fever.

3. Dry Cough

Coughing is another common symptom, but it's not just any cough. It's not a tickle in your throat. You're not just clearing your throat. It's not just irritated.

The cough is bothersome, a dry cough that you feel deep in your chest. It's coming from your breastbone or sternum, and you can tell that your bronchial tubes are inflamed or irritated.

Over 33% of 55,924 people with laboratory confirmed cases of a virus often coughed up sputum, a thick mucus sometimes called phlegm, from their lungs.

4. Chills and body aches

The beast often comes out at night: chills, body aches and high fever are often higher at night. Not everyone will have a severe reaction. Some may have no chills or body aches at all.

Others may experience milder flu-like chills, fatigue and achy joints and muscles, which can make it difficult to know if it's flu or coronavirus that's to blame.

One possible sign that you might have a virus is if your symptoms don't improve after a week or so but actually worsen.

5. Sudden confusion

Sudden confusion or an inability to wake up and be alert may be a serious sign that emergency care may be needed. If you or a loved one has those symptoms, especially with other critical signs like bluish lips, trouble breathing or chest pain, seek help immediately.

6. Digestive issues

Diarrhea or other typical gastric issues may often appear. Digestive or stomach GI (gastrointestinal) symptoms often appear.

7. Pink eye

Some people with a virus may get conjunctivitis, commonly known as pink eye.

Conjunctivitis, a highly contagious condition when caused by a virus, is an inflammation of the thin, transparent layer of tissue, called conjunctiva that covers the white part of the eye and the inside of the eyelid.

So if you have a pink or red eye, it could be one more sign that you should call your doctor if you also have other telltale symptoms, such as fever, cough or shortness of breath.

8. Loss of smell and taste

In mild to moderate cases of a virus, a loss of smell and taste is an early sign. This may be linked to loss of appetite.

Loss of smell (Anosmia) can also have causes that are not due to underlying disease. Examples include smoking, or medication side effects, or nasal obstruction, or mucus.

Anosmia, in particular, has been seen in patients ultimately testing positive for a virus with no other symptoms. It has long been known in medical literature that a sudden loss of smell may be associated with respiratory infections caused by other types of viruses.

How to test for loss of smell?

Is there anything you can do at home to test to see if you are suffering a loss of smell? The answer is yes, by using the "jellybean test" to tell if odors flow from the back of your mouth up through your nasal pharynx and into your nasal cavity. If you can pick out distinct flavors such as oranges and lemons, your sense of smell is functioning fine.

9. Fatigue

For some people, extreme fatigue can be an early sign of an illness.

Fatigue may continue long after the virus is gone. Exhaustion and lack of energy continue well past the standard recovery period of a few weeks.

10. Headache, sore throat, congestion

Many people may have headache and sore throat, and some nasal congestion, similar to colds and flu. In fact, many symptoms of a virus can resemble the flu, including headaches and the previously mentioned digestive issues, and fatigue.

Still other symptoms can resemble a cold or allergies, such as a sore throat and congestion.

However, do not be too alarmed. You simply may have a cold or the flu -- after all, they can cause fever and cough too.

How to make Penicillin

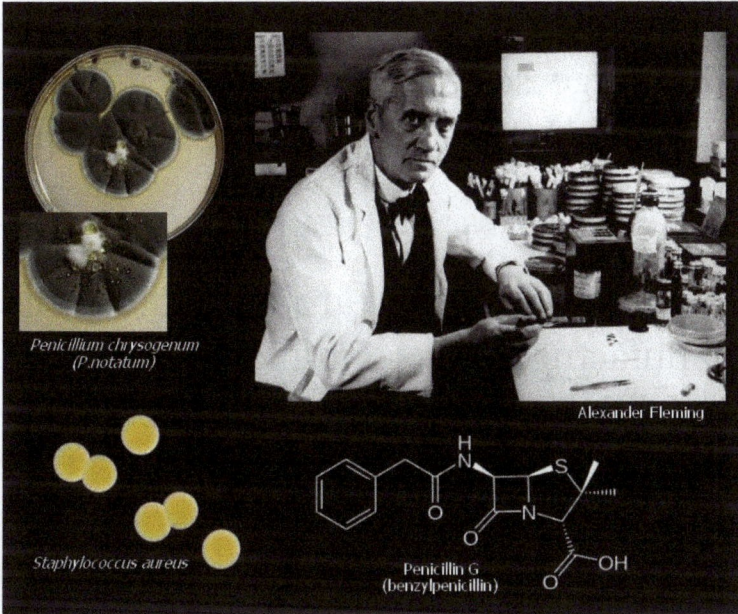

Penicillium chrysogenum
(P. notatum)

Alexander Fleming

Staphylococcus aureus

Penicillin G
(benzylpenicillin)

World War II saw major advances in medical technology including the mass production of penicillin. On March 15, 1942, U.S. made-penicillin was used to successfully treat the first patient for septicemia, blood poisoning.

This one treatment alone exhausted half of the available supply of penicillin in the United States, so the need for better techniques for produce penicillin rapidly on a large scale was necessary to help treat and U.S. soldiers fighting in Europe.

Scientists working around the clock manufactured 2.4 million doses of penicillin in preparation for the D-Day landings alone, on June 6, 1944.

Discovery

Sir Alexander Fleming discovered the bacteria-killing properties of penicillin while conducting research at St. Mary's Hospital in London in the late 1920s.

Upon returning to his disorganized lab from a weekend vacation, Fleming noticed that one of the Petri dishes was uncovered and a blue-green mold was growing inside. Rather than tossing the contaminated dish into the trash, he looked carefully and observed that the mold had killed bacteria growing nearby. Quite by accident Fleming had discovered penicillin, the antibiotic released by the mold of the genus Penicillium. Alexander Fleming was familiar with the treatment of bacterial infections after spending World

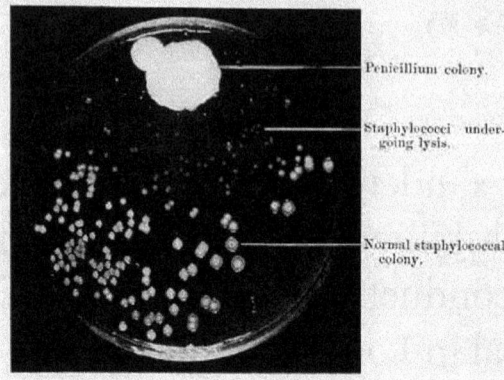

Penicillium colony.

Staphylococci under-going lysis.

Normal staphylococcal colony.

Fleming's original photograph of the contaminated dish.

In War I as a captain in the British Medical Corps. Fleming saw firsthand the lack of medicine to treat infections, with disease causing approximately one third of military deaths during the Great War. Despite its historical significance, Fleming's discovery of penicillin in 1928 brought little attention. The technology and funding needed to isolate and produce the antibiotic was unavailable at the time.

Fleming, however, continued to grow the Penicillium notatum strain in his lab for twelve years, distributing it to scientists and saving the specimen for someone willing and able to transform the "mold juice" into a medicine suitable for human use.

Purification and Trials

Meanwhile, Australian scientist Howard Florey hired Ernst Chain to help with his microbiology research at Oxford University. Florey and Chain were interested in Alexander Fleming's work and in 1938, began studying the antibacterial properties of mold. Chain began by purifying and concentrating the penicillin "juice" through a complex and tiring process of freeze drying the product repeatedly. This slow and relatively inefficient process was improved upon by another researcher, Norman Heatley, who purified the penicillin by adjusting the acidity, or pH.

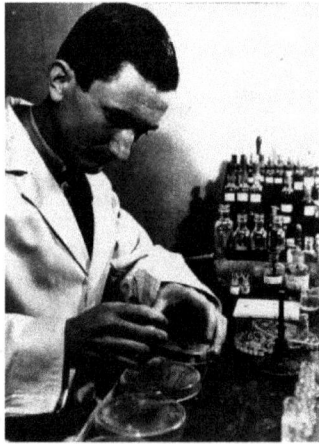

Norman Heatley working with Penicillium cultures. Photograph William Dunn School of Pathology, University of Oxford.

To their great excitement, Florey's team successfully cured infected mice with penicillin on May 25, 1940. Heatley oversaw the trials and recorded in his diary, "After supper with some friends, I returned to the lab and met the professor to give a final dose of penicillin to two of the mice.

The 'controls' were looking very sick, but the two treated mice seemed very well. I stayed at the lab until 3:45am, by which time all four control animals were dead." Delirious with excitement, Heatley returned home early that morning, surprised to find that he had put his underpants on backwards in the dark! The usually mild-mannered Heatley noted in his journal:

"It really looks as if penicillin may be of practical importance."

Mass Production

Florey and Chain's report about the mouse trials drew great interest from both scientific and military communities.

World War II was well underway in Europe and the ability to combat disease and infection could mean the difference between victory and defeat. Because British facilities were manufacturing other drugs needed for the war effort in Europe, Florey and Heatley travelled to the U.S. in July of 1941 to continue research and seek help from the American pharmaceutical industry. They convinced four drug companies, Merck, E. R. Squibb & Sons, Charles Pfizer & Co., and Lederle Laboratories, to aid in the production of penicillin.

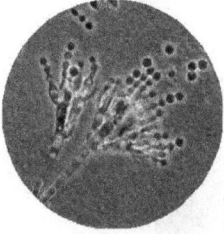

Penicillium notatum viewed with a microscope, 400x.

Florey and Heatley ended up in Peoria, Illinois to work with researchers who had perfected the fermentation process necessary for growing penicillin. The researchers in Peoria used corn instead of glucose, or simple sugar, as the nutrient source, and the penicillin grew approximately 500 times more than it had in England!

The team searched for more productive strains of Penicillium notatum, finding the best specimen growing on an over-ripe cantaloupe in a Peoria grocery store.

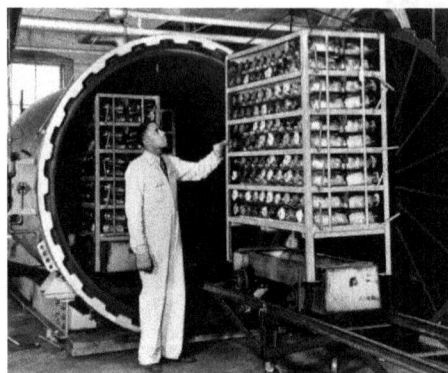

Penicillin production at pharmaceutical company, Eli Lilly.

Meanwhile, penicillin was used to cure the first human bacterial infection, proving to researchers the vital importance of the drug to save lives. But, that one cure used up the entire supply of penicillin in the entire U.S! Following Japan's attack on Pearl Harbor on December 7, 1941, it was clear to scientists and military strategists that a combined effort was needed to produce the large amounts of penicillin needed to win the war. A total of 21 U.S. companies joined together, producing 2.3 million doses of penicillin in preparation of the D-Day invasion of Normandy. Penicillin quickly became known as the war's "miracle drug," curing infectious disease and saving millions of lives.

In 1945, Sir Alexander Fleming, Ernst Chain, Sir Howard Florey were awarded the Nobel Prize in Physiology or Medicine "for the discovery of penicillin and its curative effect in various infectious diseases." We have modern antibiotics today because scientists and drug companies worked together to solve a problem.

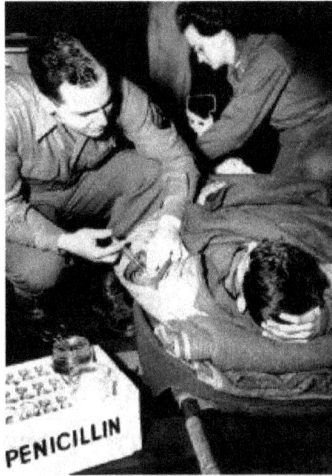

Medics using penicillin to combat infections in soldiers

Infection is always a killer, and while some soap and water could prevent it externally, but when the infection becomes inside humans, then we are often very helpless. And most anti-bacterial agent injected into the body would kill a human more quickly than the infection would.

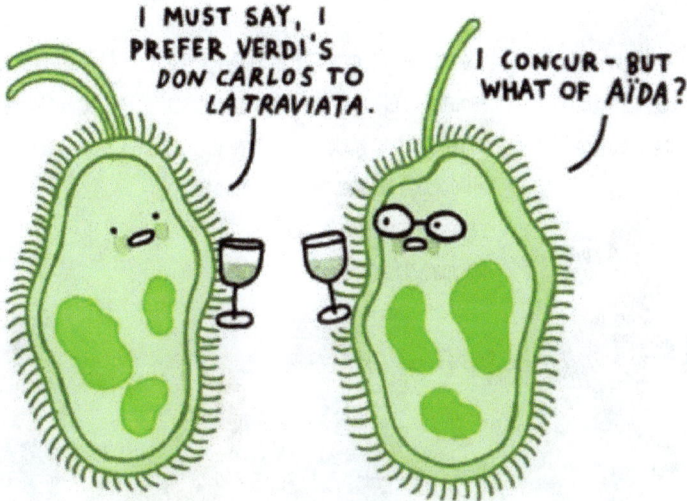

CULTURED BACTERIA

FOR MANY YEARS, scientists knew that certain molds killed some bacteria. However, researchers needed to understand how to harness this antibacterial microbe and to manufacture enough of the substance before they could make a useful medicine.

1. *Penicillium* mold naturally produces the antibiotic penicillin

2. Scientists learned to grow *Penicillium* mold in deep fermentation tanks by adding a kind of sugar and other ingredients. This process increased the growth of *Penicillium*.

3. Then, scientists separated the penicillin product from the mold.

4. Finally, penicillin is purified for use as an antibiotic medicine.

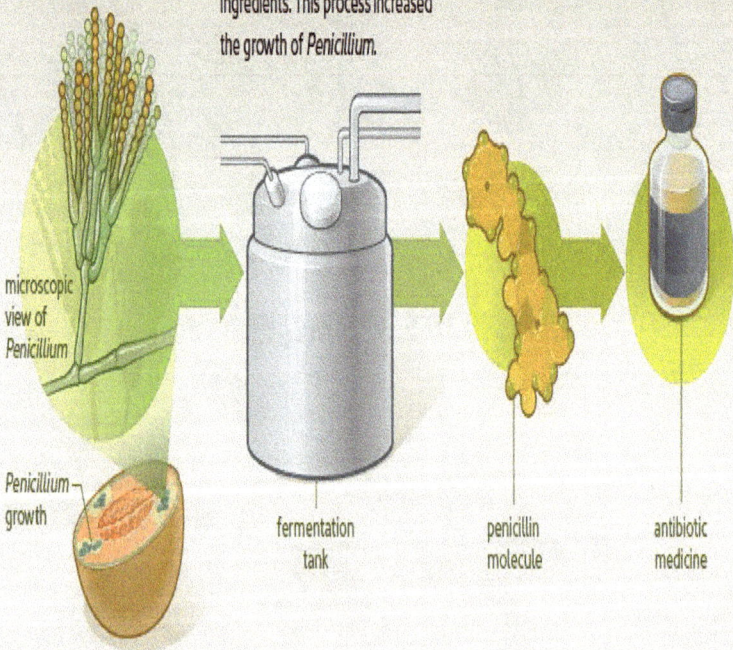

microscopic view of *Penicillium*

Penicillium growth

fermentation tank

penicillin molecule

antibiotic medicine

The rest of the book shows you how to make Penicillin Correctly with a simple Formula.

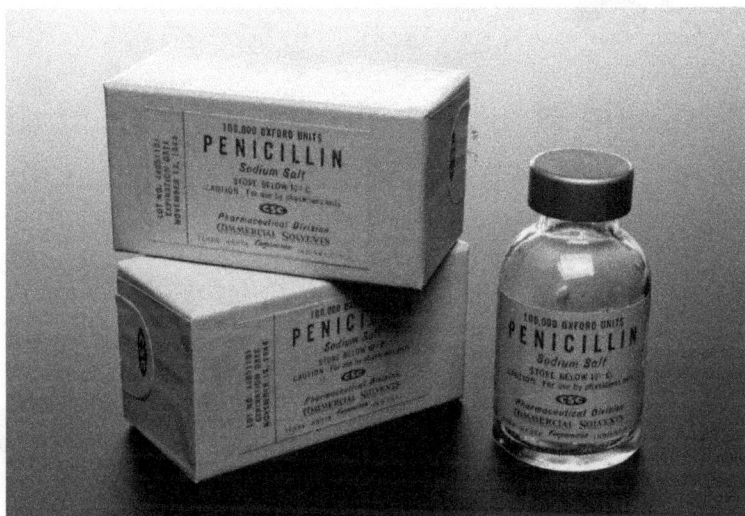

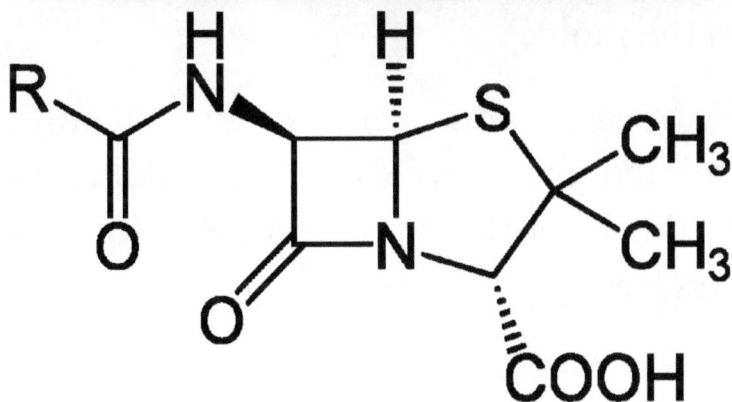

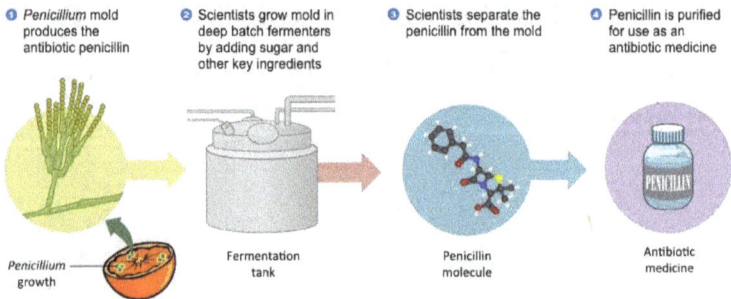

1. *Penicillium* mold produces the antibiotic penicillin
2. Scientists grow mold in deep batch fermenters by adding sugar and other key ingredients
3. Scientists separate the penicillin from the mold
4. Penicillin is purified for use as an antibiotic medicine

Penicillium growth

Fermentation tank

Penicillin molecule

Antibiotic medicine

Penicillin is an antibiotic that is used to fight pathogenic bacteria in the human body. Penicillin was truly the beginning of the antibiotic age. It was discovered in 1928, by the researcher Alexander Fleming. He figured out that bacteria in a simple petri dish that was full of Staphylococcus colonies could not grow in the mold.

However, after Alexander Fleming isolated the source from the mold, the medical world was changed for the better.

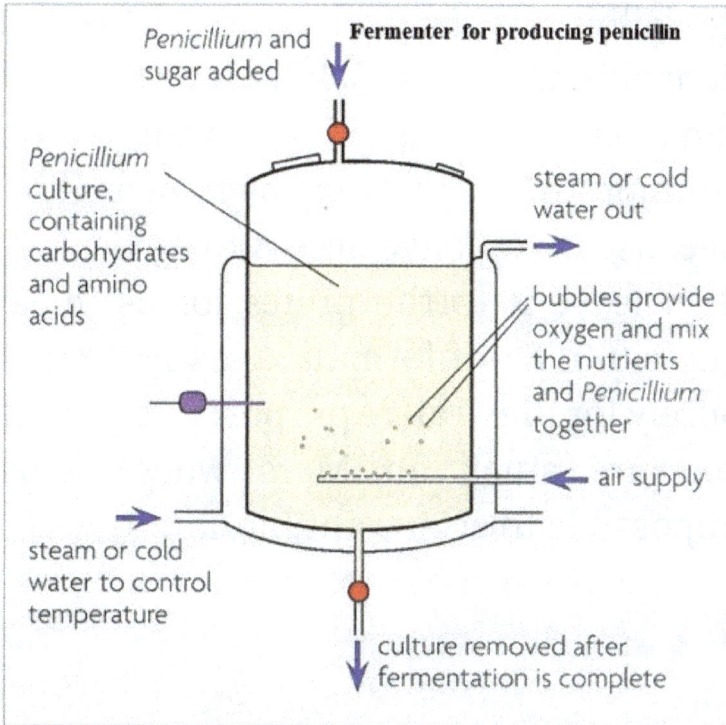

Fermenter for producing penicillin

Penicillium and sugar added

Penicillium culture, containing carbohydrates and amino acids

steam or cold water out

bubbles provide oxygen and mix the nutrients and Penicillium together

air supply

steam or cold water to control temperature

culture removed after fermentation is complete

Because of Alexander Fleming, doctors woere able to treat conditions such as pneumonia and rheumatic fever.

Pneumonia and rheumatic fever killed millions of people because of the lack of medical supplies that were affective.

Penicillin is a simply a byproduct of the Penicillium fungus. Believe it or not, you can make it at home. But you should not attempt to make your own penicillin. Because if you have access to a hospital, then leave it to the professionals make Penicillin. The information in this book is purely for illustrative purposes, such as if you are stuck on Mars where it is impossible to access antibiotics.

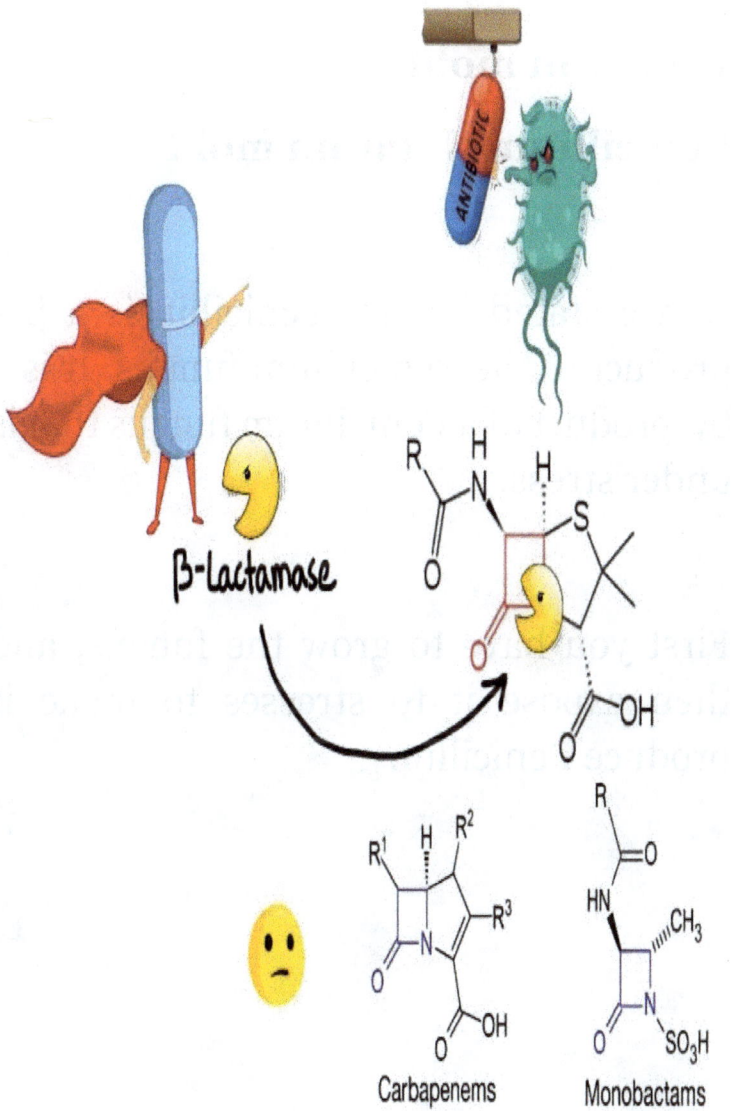

β-Lactamase

Carbapenems

Monobactams

THE FORMULA FOR PENICILLIN

Penicillin mold

Penicillium Notatum mold

As we stated before, Penicillin is a by-product of the Penicillium fungus. It is a by-product of a Penicillium fungus that is under stress.

First you have to grow the fungus, and then expose it to stresses to make it produce Penicillin.

First you need to produce a **culture** of the penicillium fungus.

A microbiological culture is simply a way of reproducing a microscopic organism by letting them reproduce in a certain environment under controlled conditions.

STEP 1

First try to expose a slice of bread or citrus peel or even a cantaloupe rind to the air in a very dark place at 70 degrees F, until a bluish-green mold develops.

Now cut two fresh slices of whole wheat bread into ½ inch cubes. Place the cubes in a 750 ml Erlenmeyer flask with a non-absorbent plug.

Note: A lot of bakeries put a substance called a mold inhibitor on their bread. This mold inhibitor will suppress fungal growth. Therefore, you must use bread that you baked yourself.

Now you must sterilize the flask and its contents in a pressure cooker for at least 20 minutes at 15 psi.

Another, method is to place it in an oven at 315 degrees Fahrenheit for one hour.

In a sterile fashion, now you must transfer the fungus from the bread or fruit peel into our flask that has our bread cubes.

Now allow the cubes to sit in a very dark place at 70 degrees F for about 5 days. This is what we call incubation. This is the easy part.

STEP 2

Now here is where it gets very complicated. You must prepare one liter of the following liquid solution:

Lactose Monohydrate	44.0 gm
Corn Starch	25.0 gm
Sodium Nitrate	3.0 gm
Magnesium Sulfate	0.25 gm
Potassium MonoPhosphate	0.50 gm
Glucose Monohydrate	2.75 gm
Zinc Sulfate	0.044 gm
Manganese Sulfate	0.044 gm

The above simple ingredients can always be found at many chemical supply houses, but you have to buy a significant amount.

Now dissolve all the ingredients in the order listed above in 500ml of cold tap water. Once you are done, then add more cold water to complete a liter (1000 ml).

After you have added the water, you must adjust the pH to 5.0-5.5 using HCL (hydrochloric acid). Here, you will need a simple pH test kit. You can find at a pet shop or most garden supply stores.

Next, you must fill glass containers with a quantity of this solution. Make sure that you use enough so that when the container is placed on its side our liquid will not touch the plug.

Next sterilize the containers and the solution in a pressure cooker or stove as we did before. Now when it cools, scrape up approximately a tablespoon of the fungus from our bread cubes and throw it into the solution.

Now you must allow the containers to incubate on their sides at 70 degrees F for about seven days.

It is very important that they are not moved around. Now if you did it correctly, you will have Penicillin in the liquid portion of the media.

Now simply filter the mixture through a coffee filter, or a thin cloth, or something similar, then plug the bottle containers, and refrigerate them immediately.

STEP 3

How to extract our penicillin from the solution:

Simply adjust the cold solution to pH 2.2 using (.01 %) HCL. Then mix it with cold ethyl acetate in a **separatory funnel** (this is a funnel with a stopcock, you can find most or all these items at chemistry glass suppliers) and shake well for about 30 seconds or so.

Now drain the ethyl acetate, which is on the bottom, into a clean beaker which has been placed in an ice bath and repeat the process.

Now add 1% potassium acetate and mix well. We want the ethyl acetate to evaporate off.

This can be done or induced by a constant flow of air over the top of the beaker, like from a fan. Wait until it dries. The remaining crystals are simply a mixture of potassium penicillin and potassium acetate.

That is it! You just built a simple laboratory and made you have truly made Penicillin!

Now you are the mad scientist that just made Penicillin!

Foods that Fights Respiratory and Fungal Infections

Fungal infections forms: *candida, athletes foot, yeast infection.* Starving the yeast is the best way to treat fungal infections.

Fungi are primitive organisms and are everywhere in our environment such as in our air, in the soil, even on plants and in water. We see Fungi almost every day, such as mildew, mold. Mushrooms are a form of fungi too.

In the woman's vagina, a candida infection is commonly known as a yeast infection.

People with diabetes get yeast infections often. Vinegar and Apple cider vinegar are a scientifically proven antifungal. Laboratory research shows that it can inhibit the growth of candida cultivating in a petri dish.

I also recommend adding a tea spoon of Apple Cider to your bird's or parrot's water dish. And like humans, cats and dogs do not like vinegar much, but it is good for them. Add a spoon of Apple Cider each day to their fresh water bowl. Add Apple Cider only once a day, but change the water bowl twice a day, so pets that are sensitive to vinegar are not harmed.

If fungi and yeast is everywhere, then why humans are not sick all the time? This is because only half of all types of fungi are very harmful, but the other half is perfectly benign.

While oral antifungal and topical medications are often necessary, the food we eat can often prevent or treat fungal infections. Many plant and foods have fungal fighting properties such as anti-parasitic, anti-microbial, and anti-bacterial agents.

Foods that have high fungal fighting properties include:

- Vinegar
- Apple cider vinegar
- Garlic
- Onion
- Coconut oil
- Ginger
- Pumpkin seeds
- Cinnamon, cloves
- Lemons and Lime

Next I will present many food recipes that will incorporate these all the natural fungus-fighting foods.

1. Crispy Rice with Coconut Oil

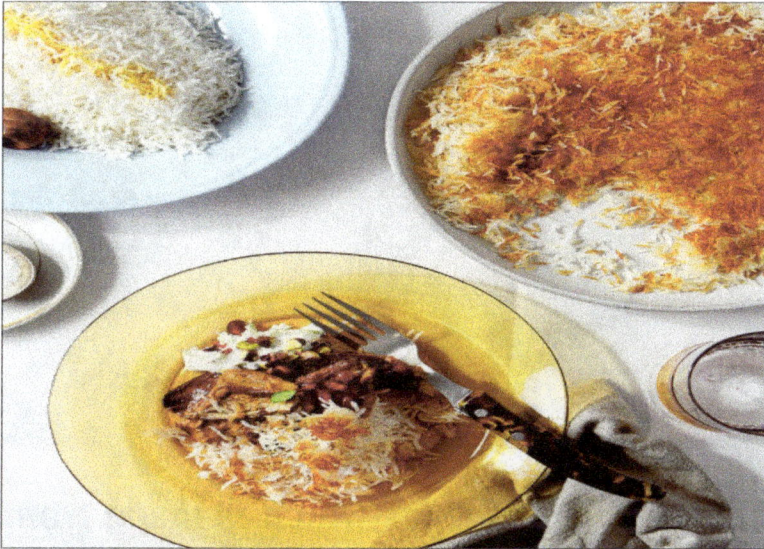

Coconut Oil and products fights off fungal infections. Coconut oil has strong antifungal and antibacterial properties. It fights off fungal infections such as yeast and candida infections. This Crispy Rice with Coconut Oil dish uses 3 tablespoons of fungus fighting coconut oil.

2. Muffins with Apple Cider

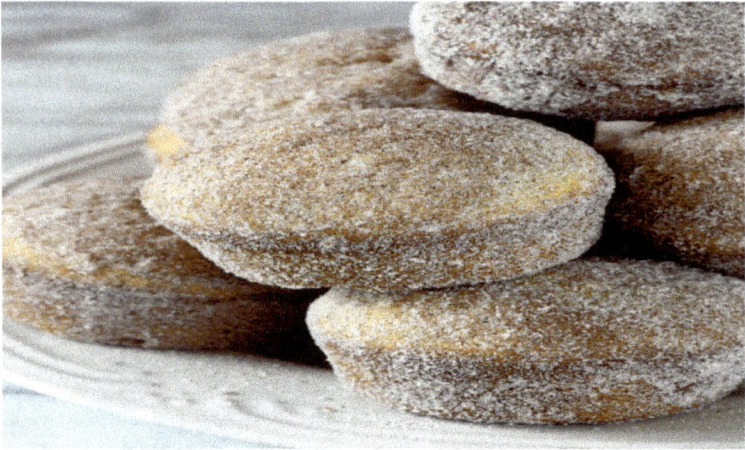

Apple cider vinegar which is made from crushed, aged, and fermented apples is great for all sorts of cuisines and due to its colonies of good bacteria, it can also be used as a body cleanser. Apple cider vinegar is a strong and effective fungus killer. These Muffins with Apple Cider has 1/3 cup of apple cider vinegar, combined with fungus fighting cinnamon. Use coconut oil instead of canola oil and you have a powerful fungus fighting treat.

3. Blistered Shishitos with Ginger plus Garlic

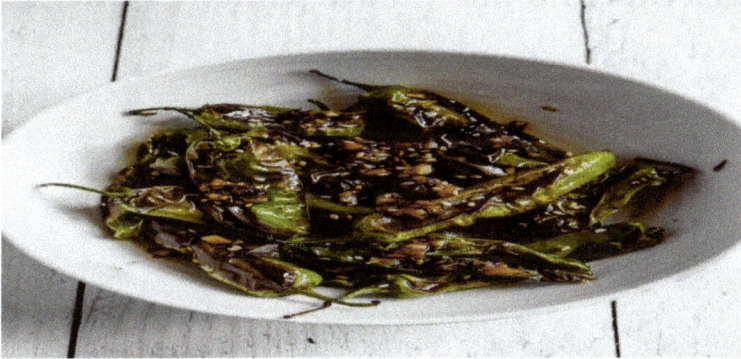

Ginger and garlic have strong antibacterial and antifungal properties. Ginger and garlic have been used since Jesus's time as natural remedies for many ailments. Allicin is a compound produced when garlic is crushed or chopped. It has a very potent antibiotic quality. Ginger which is often used to treat nausea, also has antifungal properties. These Blistered Shishito Peppers with Ginger and Garlic are easy to make and can make a wonderful treat.

Along with the garlic cloves and minced ginger, add fresh lime juice and healthy olive oil and fat-filled sesame.

4. Coconut Kaffir Lime Cooler

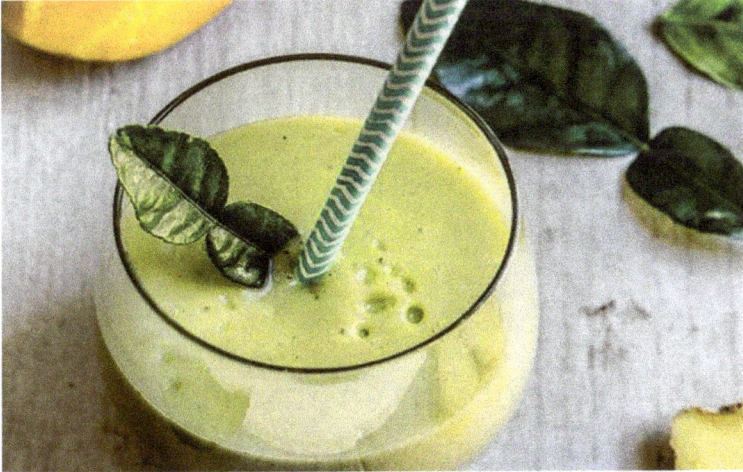

Packing a powerful antifungal one-two punch, this Coconut Kaffir Lime Cooler calls for two coconut-rich products — milk and water — along with a dose of fresh antifungal and antibacterial ginger. This beverage infuses the nutrients together with a bit of citrus and the sweet tang of fresh mango!

5. Garlic Miso and Onion Soup

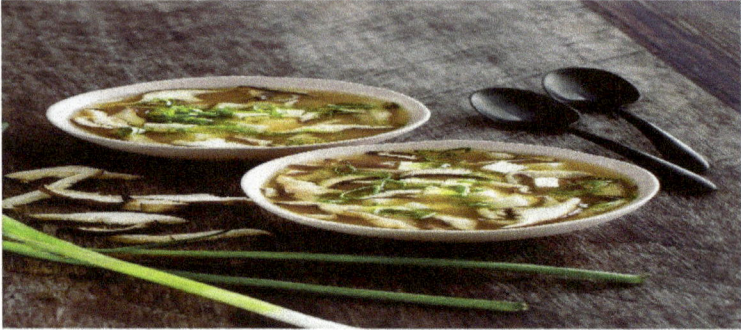

Onions are not only an aromatic pleasure and flavor enhancer, but they also have antifungal, antibacterial, and antiparasitic properties. Plus, onions also "help the kidneys to flush excess fluids out the body," keeping sodium and water levels balanced in the body. This Garlic Miso and Onion Soup calls for one and a half onions, four whole cloves of garlic, and a half of a cup of shiitake mushrooms, all of which are great for fighting fungal infections. In addition, this soup uses protein-rich tofu, fermented miso and soy sauce, and healthy fat-filled sesame oil.

6. Homemade Pumpkin Seed Milk

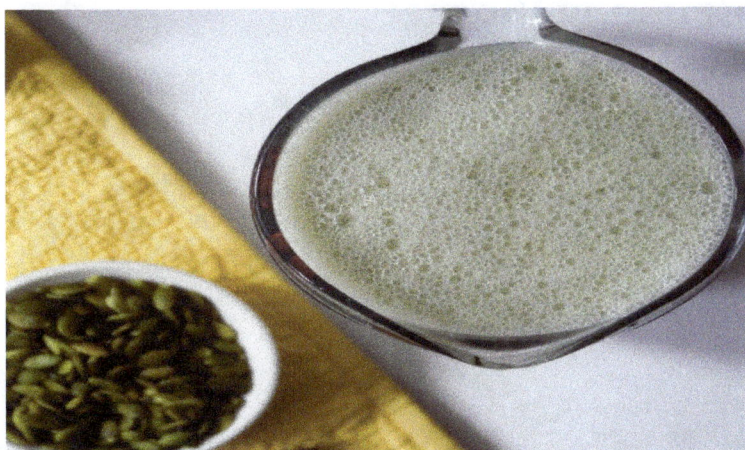

Seeds are a staple in any plant-based diet as they are usually high in fat and other essential nutrients. Pumpkin seeds are no exception! They are high in omega-3 fatty acids, plus these tasty seeds "have antifungal, antiviral and anti-parasitic properties." This Homemade Pumpkin Seed Milk is a rich and tasty source of pumpkin seeds! The recipe calls for a full cup of pumpkin seeds and adds a warming flavor with nutmeg, dates, and vanilla extract.

7. Rhubarb and Ginger Shrub Drinking Vinegar

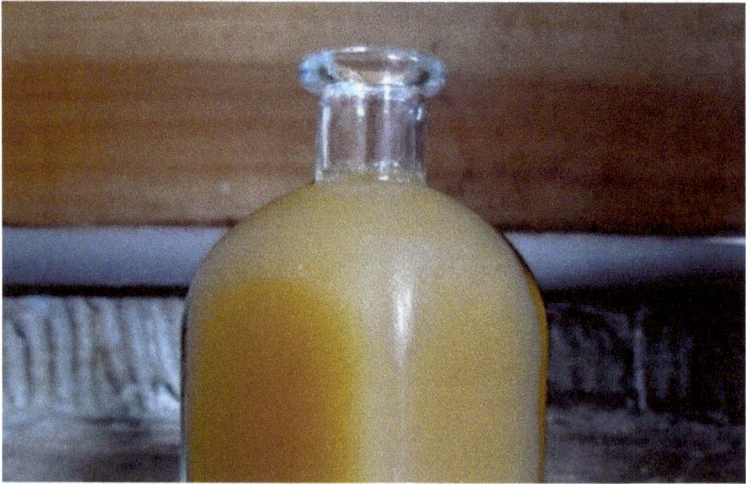

While apple cider vinegar is excellent for baking sweet treats, it can also be used to give beverages a spicy-sweet kick of flavor! This Rhubarb and Ginger Shrub Drinking Vinegar calls for fungus-fighting a full cup of apple cider vinegar and two tablespoons of fresh ginger.

8. Cinnamon and Clove Mixed Nut and Seed Milk

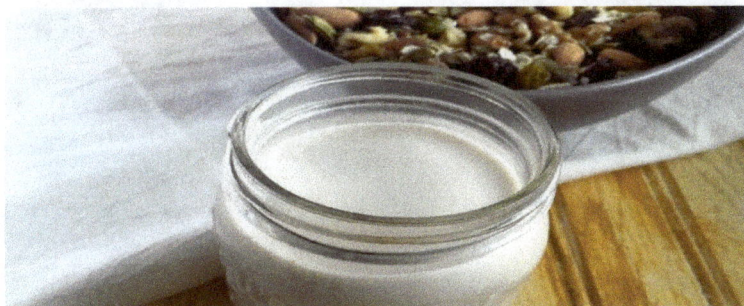

Cinnamon and cloves offer two ends of the spice spectrum — one being warm, spicy, and sweet, while the other is earthy, nutty, and rich. As different as their flavors are, both of these spices are great for fighting fungal infections. Cinnamon "has been used as an anti-inflammatory and anticancer agent," while cloves have a variety of antifungal and immune system stimulating constituents. This Cinnamon and Clove Mixed Nut and Seed Milk calls for both cinnamon and cloves, along with a host of nutrient-dense nuts and seeds.

9. Cinnamon Linseed Pancakes

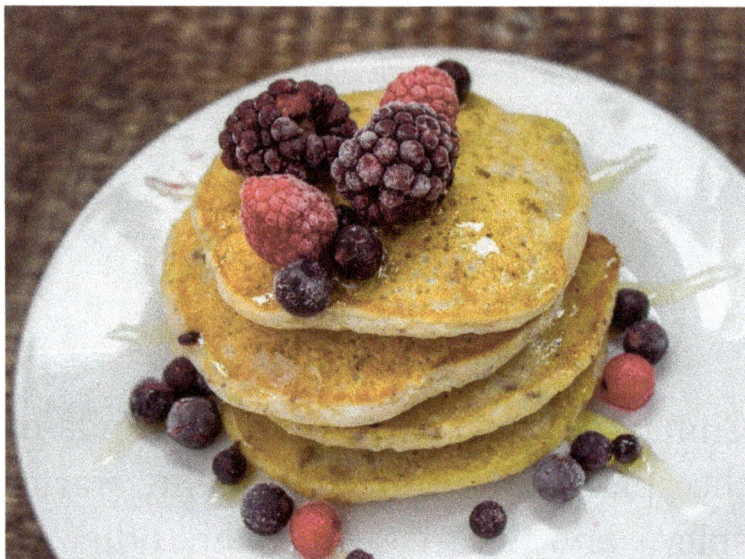

Looking for a warm and tasty recipe to get your body going in the morning? These Cinnamon Linseed Pancakes not only will boost your digestion for the day with a helping of fiber-rich linseed (also known as flaxseed), but it also uses fungus-fighting cinnamon and coconut oil!

10. Lemon Sautéed Asparagus

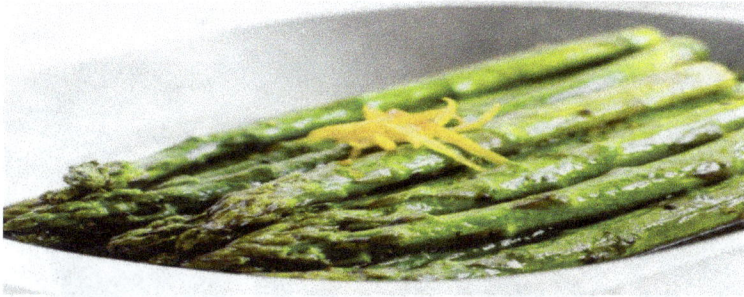

Lemon juice is rich in essential nutrients — such as vitamin A, vitamin C, folate, calcium, magnesium, phosphorous, and potassium — and is a good source of healthy sugars for those sweet recipes you crave. Yet, lemon juice has also been found to have anti-fungal properties, as well as "help detoxify your liver," both of which aid the body heal and fight fungal infections. This recipe calls for lemon zest — shavings of lemon rind — balancing out the sweetness of the juice, as well as healthy fat-rich olive oil.

11. Blood Orange, Carrot and Ginger Smoothie

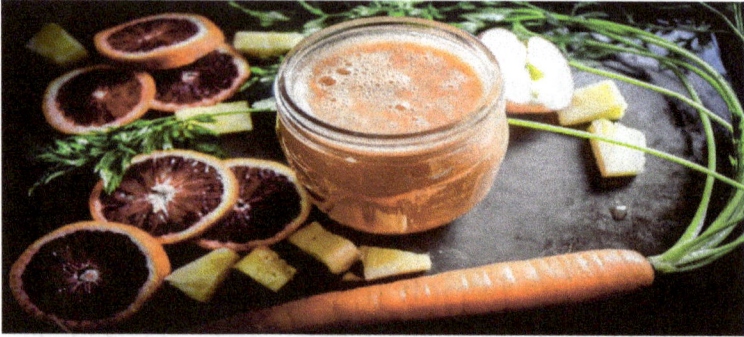

Smoothies are an excellent way to get your necessary dose of essential nutrients without a kitchen handy. This Blood Orange, Carrot and Ginger Smoothie has the added benefit of using fungus-fighting coconut milk and grated fresh ginger. Plus, the powerful mixture of antioxidants and vitamin C from the carrots and pineapple, the pectin (a unique form of fiber) from apples, and the inflammation-fighting and folic acid rich blood orange, make this the perfect smoothie to fight off ailments of any kind or simply keep a healthy body healthy!

12. Chaga Vinegar

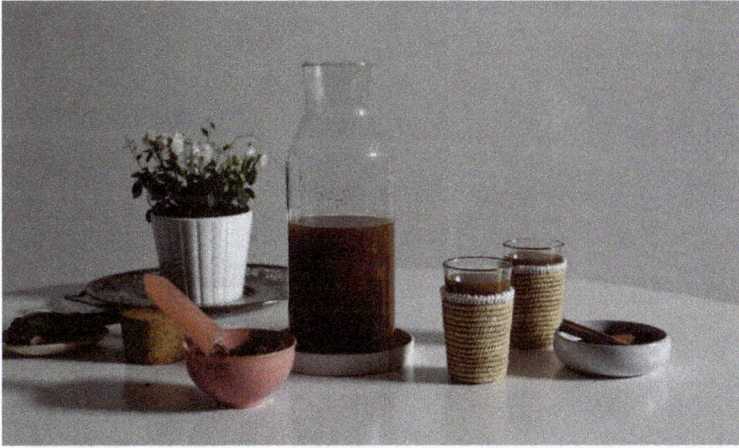

This Chaga Vinegar only has four simple ingredients: A third of a cup of adaptogenic Chaga mushrooms will help level out your body's natural stress response, lower anxiety, and provide energy. A full liter of apple cider, plus a cinnamon stick will fight fungal infections and provide a detoxifying effect. Plus, that vanilla bean has health benefits as well such as fighting acne, reducing anxiety, and promoting good digestion!

13. Patatas Bravas with Garlic Aioli

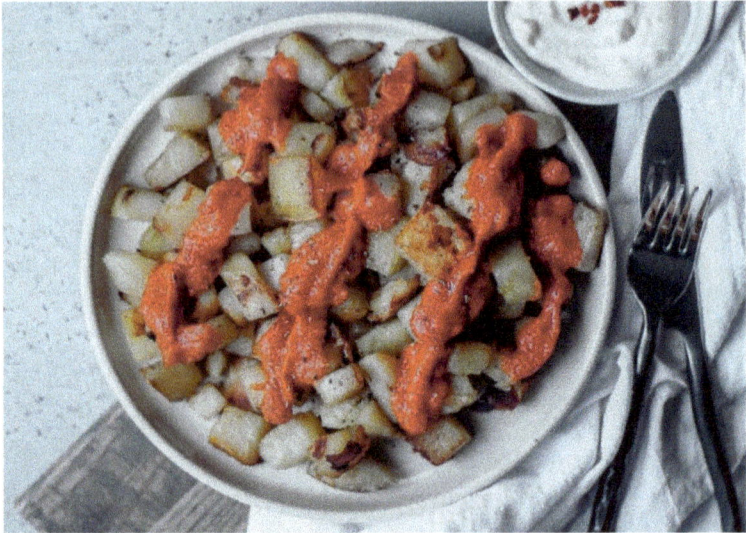

This dairy-free, vegan Patatas Bravas with Garlic Aioli recipe is a great way to get your daily dose of fungus-fighting garlic, as well as a slew of other nutrient-rich, plant-based food. This patatas bravas call for around four minced cloves of garlic, as well as fungus-fighting onions, and healthy fat-rich olive oil!

14. Coconut Oil Cookies

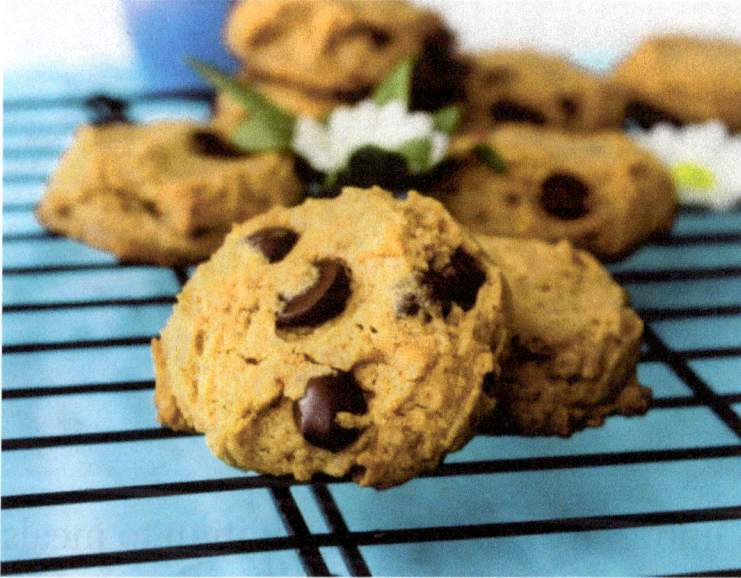

Hankering for something sweet? Instead of reaching for that pre-packaged box of cookies — filled with processed ingredients — try having these Coconut Oil Cookies on hand! They are rich in fungus-fighting coconut oil, nutrient-filled coconut sugar, and fiber-filled nuts!

15. Onion and Pepper Masala

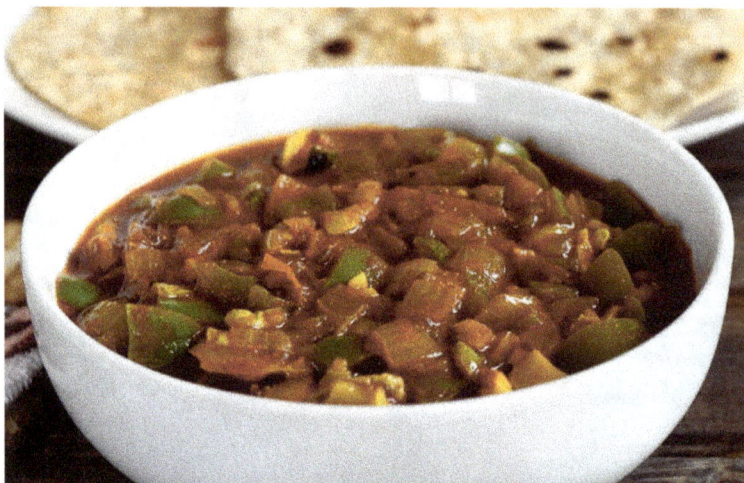

Onions are a great side addition to meals that require a bit more flavor, yet they can also be the main player! This Onion and Pepper not only favors onions — one large onion, in fact — but it also incorporates other fungus-fighting agents such as cloves, ginger, and oil of your choice (substitute coconut oil!). Plus, it incorporates other anti-inflammatory foods such as turmeric — rich in curcumin — and antioxidant-rich bell peppers.

Making Yogurt at Home for people with Diabetes

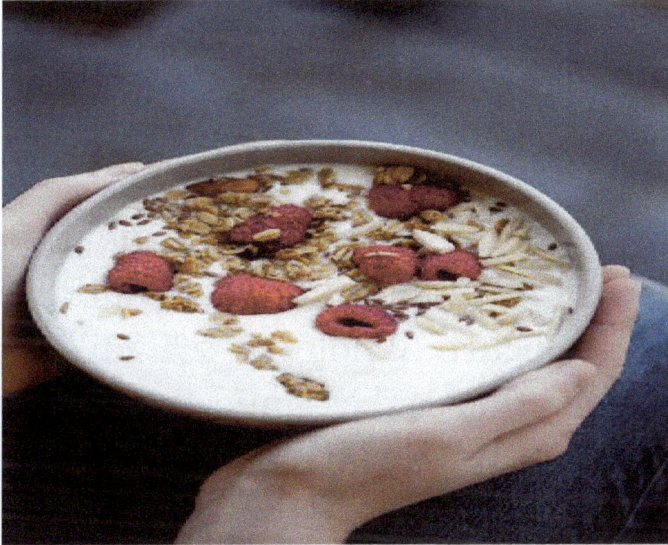

Most dairy products have a low Glycemic Index (GI). This makes them ideal for people with diabetes. Yogurts that contain a total carbohydrate content of 15 g or less per serving are ideal for people with diabetes.

Look for yogurts that are high in protein and low in carbohydrates, such as unflavored Greek yogurt.

What Do I Need to Make Yogurt?

All you need to make homemade yogurt is a half gallon of milk and about a half cup of yogurt. Whole or 2% milk will make the thickest, creamiest yogurt, but you can also use skim milk if you like. For the yogurt, either Greek or regular yogurt is fine, but avoid any flavorings; stick to plain, unflavored yogurts.

When you are buying yogurt, also check that it lists "Live Active Yogurt Cultures" in the ingredients — we need those! The live cultures are what actually turn the milk into yogurt.

The number of cultures doesn't really matter; as long as there is at least one, you can make yogurt. This said, different strains of bacteria have different health benefits, so look for the yogurt with the most number of cultures listed. Some common ones are L. Bulgaricus, S. Thermophilus, L. Acidophilus, Bifidus, L. Casei.

What Equipment Do I Need?

All you need to make yogurt is a heavy pot with a lid. You can uuse a 3-quart Dutch oven. Once the lid is on, a heavy pot like this does an admirable job of keeping the milk cozy and at a fairly steady temperature (ideally around 110°F) while the bacteria go to work turning the milk into yogurt.

It also helps to put the pot somewhere insulated and warm while this is happening, like an oven with the light turned on or a picnic cooler with a hot water bottle.

You can certainly use a yogurt maker or even a dehydrator if you have one — these are great for holding the yogurt at a very steady temperature as it incubates — but you can make great yogurt without them.

What Next?

Once you have this basic method for making yogurt down pat, there are all sorts of tweaks and changes you can make. Some people like to add dry milk powder or gelatin for extra thickness, others like to strain off the liquid whey for a dense Greek-style yogurt.

Using different brands of commercial yogurt to culture the milk can also give you subtly different flavors and nutritional benefits. You can also try purchasing a special starter from a health food store, food co-op or online. My favorite resource for interesting starters is Cultures for Health.

Making 2 quarts of yogurt

INGREDIENTS

8 cups milk (1/2 gallon) — whole or 2% are best, but skim can also be used

1/2 cup commercial yogurt containing active cultures

EQUIPMENT

- 3 quart or larger Dutch oven or heavy saucepan with a lid

- Spatula
- Instant-read or candy thermometer (one that can clip to the side of the pan)
- Small measuring cup or small bowl
- Whisk

INSTRUCTIONS

Heat the milk. Pour the milk into a Dutch oven and place over medium to medium-high heat. Warm the milk to right below boiling, about 200°F. Stir the milk gently as it heats to make sure the bottom doesn't scorch and the milk doesn't boil over. According to the National Center for Home Food Preservation, this heating step is necessary to change the protein structure in the milk so it sets as a solid instead of separating.

Cool the milk. Let the milk cool until it is just warm to the touch, 112°F to 115°F. Stir occasionally to prevent a skin from forming. (Though if one does form, you can either stir it back in or pull it out for a snack!) You can help this step go faster by placing the Dutch oven in an ice water bath and gently stirring the milk.

Thin the yogurt with milk. Scoop out about a cup of warm milk into a bowl. Add the yogurt and whisk until smooth and the yogurt is dissolved in the milk.

Whisk the thinned yogurt into the milk. While whisking gently, pour the thinned yogurt into the warm milk. This inoculates the milk with the yogurt culture.

Transfer the pot to the (turned-off) oven. Cover the Dutch oven and place the whole pot in a turned-off oven — turn on the oven light or wrap the pot in towels to keep the milk warm as it sets (ideally around 110°F, though some variance is fine). You can also make the yogurt in a dehydrator left at 110°F or using a yogurt maker.

Wait for the yogurt to set. Let the yogurt set for at least 4 hours or as long as overnight — the exact time will depend on the cultures used, the temperature of the yogurt, and your yogurt preferences. The longer yogurt sits, the thicker and more tart it becomes. If this is your first time making yogurt, start checking it after 4 hours and stop when it reaches a flavor and consistency you like. Avoid jostling or stirring the yogurt until it has fully set.

Cool the yogurt. Once the yogurt has set to your liking, remove it from the oven. If you see any watery whey on the surface of the yogurt, you can either drain this off or whisk it back into the yogurt before transferring to containers. Whisking also gives the yogurt a more consistent creamy texture. Transfer the to storage containers, cover, and refrigerate. Homemade yogurt will keep for about 2 weeks in the refrigerator. Your next batch of homemade yogurt. Once you start making your own yogurt, you can use some of each batch to culture your next batch. Just save 1/2 cup to use for this purpose. If after a few batches, you notice some odd flavors in your yogurt or that it's not culturing quite as quickly, that means that either some outside bacteria has taken up residence in your yogurt or that this strain is becoming weak.

As long as this batch still tastes good to you, it will be safe to eat, but go back to using some store-bought commercial yogurt in your next batch.

Holding the temperature: If your milk drops below 110°F while it's incubating, that's fine. It will take a little longer to set and might end up a little looser, but the bacteria in the yogurt culture will keep the milk from spoiling. By the way, even after 8 hours in the oven (overnight), our yogurt made in the Dutch oven still usually registers about 100°F when I take it out of the oven!

Homemade Greek yogurt: You can make Greek-style yogurt by straining your homemade yogurt until it is as thick as you like.

Virus Pandemics

Virus pandemics originate at a market selling wild animals for food, such as in China, Vietnam, Korea and other Asian countries.

God forbade humans to kill one another. God also forbade humans to kill or eat any animal that kills, or eats blood or flesh.

Feasting on exotic animals became a sign of status and wealth in many Asian countries. The desire for wildlife as food or medicine drives a trade in wild animals, some procured illegally, creating a breeding ground for disease and the chance for viruses to leap to humans.

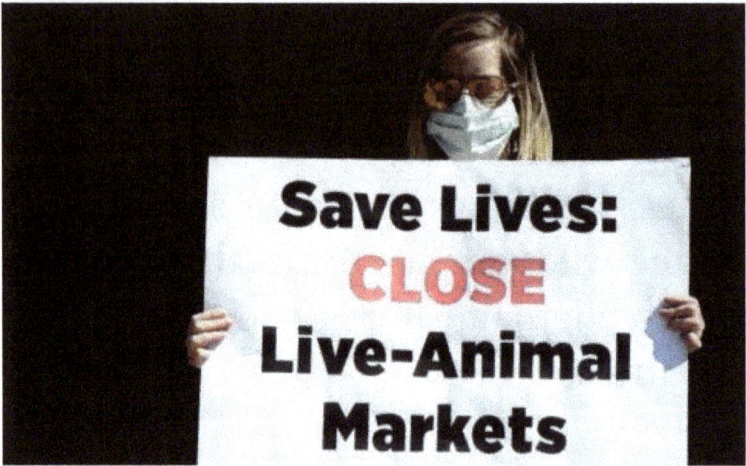

The consumption of wild animals, especially wild mammals, which can carry diseases that can cross the species barrier, does pose a real threat to human health.

Wet markets

Wet markets have become a familiar sight in many countries in Southeast Asia, particularly mainland China.

Selling live fish, chickens and wildlife, as well as fresh fruit and vegetables, they get their name from the melting ice used to preserve goods, as well as to wash the floors clean of blood from butchered animals.

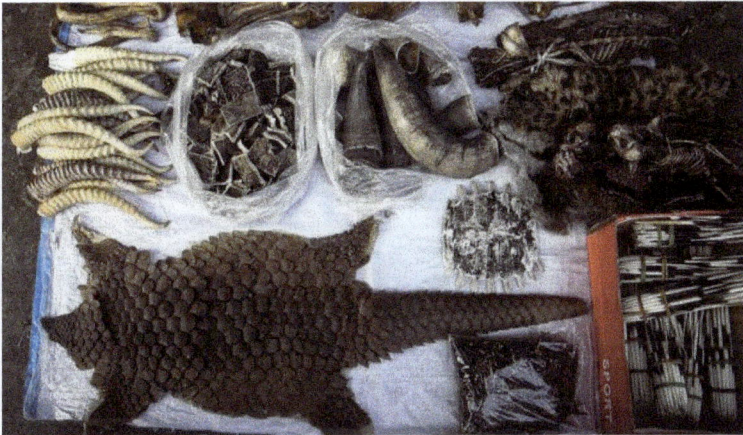

Wet markets can be "**timebombs**" for epidemics. This sort of way that we treat... animals as if they are just our commodities for us to plunder - it comes back to bite us and it's no surprise.

Leap to humans

Every few decades a virus pandemic, claims tens of thousands of lives, and almost always originates in China in their food market. These markets sell snakes, bats, porcupine, tigers, lions, deer, bears, and many other wildlife for rich Asians to eat. Such animals carry viruses which can leap to humans.

Scientists have for decades been drawing attention to outbreaks of human diseases that have originated in animals, including Severe Acute Respiratory Syndrome (Sars), Middle East Respiratory Syndrome (Mers) and Ebola.

Avoid traveling to Asia and avoid live animal markets that trade in wildlife.

Not only will this help prevent the spread of disease, it will address one of the major drivers of species extinction.

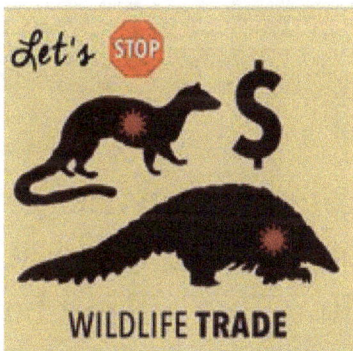

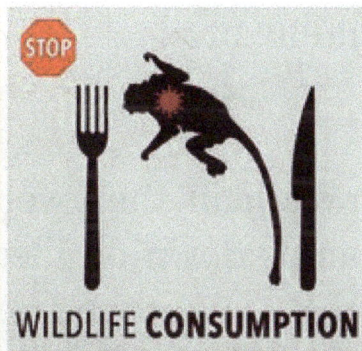

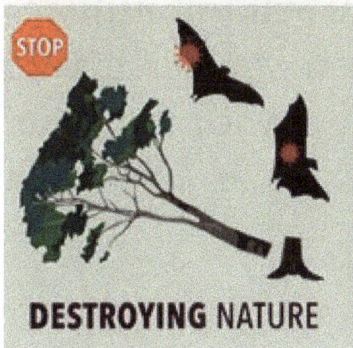

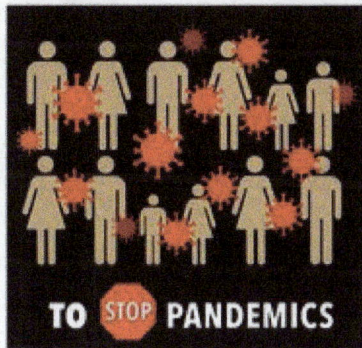

Thousands of wildlife farms raising animals such as porcupines, civets and turtles are often shut down. However, loopholes will always remain, such as the trade in wild animals for medicine, pets and scientific research.

Then there is the traditional Chinese medicines industry, which also uses wildlife products.

In Vietnam, the government often tries to clamps down on illegal wildlife trade at street markets and online. But will not be easy to change ignorant cultural attitudes or to enforce bans, when wet markets are part of the local culture, with the belief that the meat sold there is fresh and cheap.

Supply and demand

The issue is ignorant greed and demand. The people who are providing them, whether that is farmed wild animals or animals from the wild, are doing it for greed and profits.

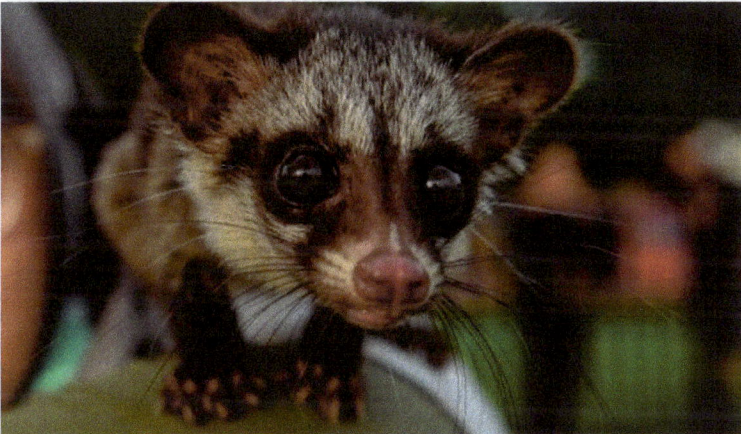

Each year the World Health Organization says that more than 15,000 lives are lost each year because they ate bats, snakes, bears, tigers, monkeys, and mongoose-like civets, and other wild animals.

To stop pandemics, we must focus on causes as well as effects. At the root of the problem is the destruction of nature, bringing animals and humans into conflict.

Even in protected forests, the forests are still there, but the wildlife's gone from within them because they have ended up in food markets. And it is easy to finger point, but it is not just happening in China, it is happening in many other countries and even in the western world. We like to have exotic pets and many of those are wild caught and we ought to be putting our own house in order too.

How to make Insulin for Diabetes

The most significant problem from diabetes, before the creation of 'human' insulin, was falling into a hyperglycemic induced coma. Before the invention of 'human' insulin, doctors were able to help some diabetics prolong their life by only as long as a year or two with very careful management of carbohydrate intake.

Before insulin, being diagnosed with diabetes meant starving to death and eventually falling into coma. Most diabetes patients were in such painfully malnourished states, and often weighing under 75 pounds upon admittance to a hospital, then death a few days or months later.

What to Know about
Diabetic Ketoacidosis (DKA)

DKA is a serious condition that can result from untreated or undiagnosed diabetes or from too little insulin. It can lead to a diabetic coma or even death.

EARLY SIGNS OF DKA

Feeling very thirsty

Urinating often

High blood glucose levels

High ketone levels in urine

LATER, EXTREME SIGNS

Feeling weak or constantly sleepy

Dry/flushed skin

Nausea, vomiting, pain in the abdomen

Difficulty breathing, fruity-smelling breath

KNOW THE SIGNS,
SAVE LIVES.

Learn more about diabetic ketoacidosis and appropriate emergency treatment at **diabetes.org/dka.**

⚠ If you think you have diabetic ketoacidosis, contact your doctor IMMEDIATELY, or go to the nearest hospital emergency room.

American Diabetes Association.

It is difficult to have diabetes, especially because the person is insulin dependent. Even nowadays, when most people have no health insurance and limited access to health care. A careful management of carbohydrate intake is important, but If Shit Hits The Fan, knowing how to make insulin can make the difference between life and death.

Type 1 diabetes is a very tricky illness that always needs a very special diet and also constant medication, i.e. insulin. In some disaster scenario, a person with diabetes is much more vulnerable than others.

When a person have diabetes, they are playing a nonstop game with their body trying to stay alive. First, the diabetic person is insulin dependent. Moreover, the person is much more prone to various infections and illnesses.

I have more than just a passing interest in chemistry and finding a way to beat diabetes. Most of my family died from heart disease or stroke due to diabetes. My kid daughter too suffered a diabetic coma and died before her 5th birthday. She was such a young kid. Not even one 5 years old. She had a fever for two days, a cough, and diarrhea. The fever had gone on for more than any other kind of cold a baby gets. Something was truly wrong.

I held my daughter in my arms all nights. I would fall asleep on the chair holding her or I would not sleep at all. One night, she stopped crying. She was silent, and less responsive and she started breathing funny. My wife jumped up and quickly called our pediatrician and told her what was happening. The doctor then asked my wife to put the phone up to her mouth so she could hear her breathing.

It has been over 20 years, and I can still remember her sweet smell. I can also still remember the doctor yelling. I could hear her, over the phone, despite being on the other side of the kitchen. "Take her to the hospital now! I will meet you there and I will call ahead so that they know that you are coming!" She then hung up.

This left us very stunned and shaking. I remember my wife looking at me very confused with tears streaming down her face as she was collecting things to take. Just as we were about to leave, the phone rang. I answered it. "You have not left yet?" "No, we are still getting her stuff together." "Then hurry the hell up!" And then she hung up again. I did not say anything to my wife. She was crying and going as fast as lightening.

Then off we went. The nurses told us a few days later that the doctors were lost and struggled to make the diagnosis.

The doctor came out and said, "She is dying, and I do not know why. I have just called a specialist doctor, a good friend, for help. We will keep an eye on her until she is gone."

Quickly the specialist had the bright idea to treat her elevated blood sugars.

My daughter went from death's door, and I honestly mean, right from the edge of death's door, to smiling in just 24 hours. It was Diabetic ketoacidosis (DKA). She was diabetic.

DKA is an acute, major, life-threatening complication of diabetes that mainly occurs in patients with type 1 diabetes, however, it is not uncommon in some patients with type 2 diabetes.

It was not until a few years later that I put all the pieces together as to why it took so long to diagnose my beautiful daughter with simple DKA. My daughter, unlike most patients with diabetes, went into DKA at a relatively very low blood sugar– somewhere in the 160 range, instead of the 400 to 900 range, beyond normal, that send most patients with diabetes over the edge. Prolonged blood sugar extremes — blood sugar that is either too high or too low for too long — may cause various conditions, all of which can lead to a diabetic coma

Now fast forward about 5 years later. One day I was coming to the apartment for lunch. I walked into a quiet apartment. My wife was sleeping on the couch. I took my jacket off and I walked into the kitchen. There at the table I saw my beautiful daughter, with blood running down all her fingers and dripping on the table.

In a loud voice, I said, "What happened?" She turned towards me with those brown, beautiful watery eyes towards me, and, her lips trembling, she said, "I did not want to wake mom up, and I was dizzy and wanted to learn how to check my blood sugar." I snatched her up and held her so tight; both of us cried much.

She cried from her broken fingers, and I cried from a broken and tired heart.

She was still so tiny and young. She had the knowledge and coordination to poke her tiny finger with the lancet device, but she still lacked the coordination to get the drop of blood on the meter's strip. So she had stuck the next finger, and then the next finger, until all fingers and even her tiny thumb were dripping blood. I am not sure if she was crying from fear or pain, because by that time for certain her fingertips had lost all sensations. It was a shattering day for me. I was much more devastated the day that I lost her forever.

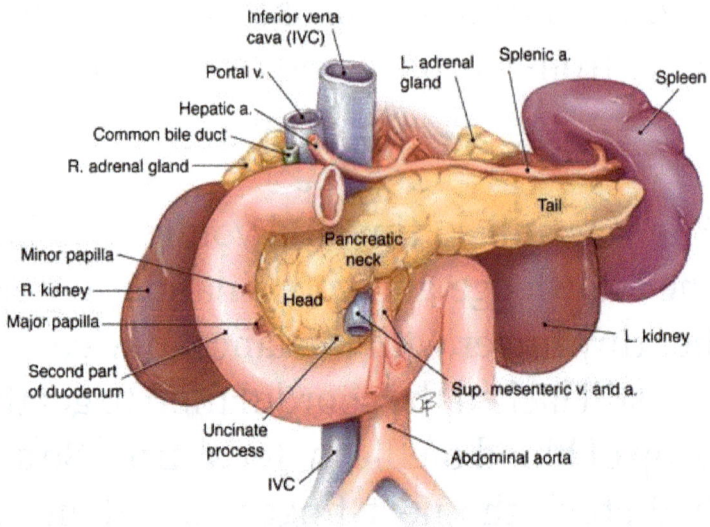

Inferior vena cava (IVC)

L. adrenal gland

Splenic a.

Spleen

Portal v.

Hepatic a.

Common bile duct

R. adrenal gland

Tail

Minor papilla

Pancreatic neck

R. kidney

Head

Major papilla

L. kidney

Second part of duodenum

Sup. mesenteric v. and a.

Uncinate process

Abdominal aorta

IVC

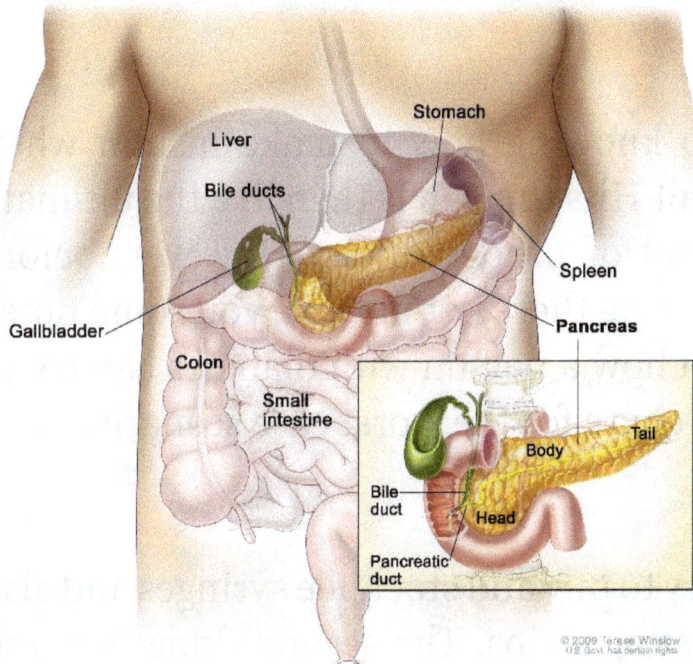

Liver

Stomach

Bile ducts

Spleen

Gallbladder

Pancreas

Colon

Small intestine

Bile duct

Body

Tail

Head

Pancreatic duct

© 2009 Terese Winslow
U.S. Govt. has certain rights

When Shit Hits the Fan

So knowing how to make insulin when Shit Hits the Fan is then like the ultimate level of preparedness. However, before getting there, let me give you some notes on how a person with diabetes can try to prepare for the worst case scenario.

Try to buy and stockpile syringes and also testing strips. The second thing that you will need is insulin. Insulin that is not in use should be stored in the refrigerator, but never freeze. If refrigeration is not possible, it can be kept at room temperature [15-25 degrees Celsius, or 59-77 Fahrenheit] for 28 days. Please keep in mind that expired insulin will kill you (expired insulin forms crystals that are lethal when injected).

Insulin is very sensitive to sunlight, indoor lights, and to extremely hot or cold temperature.

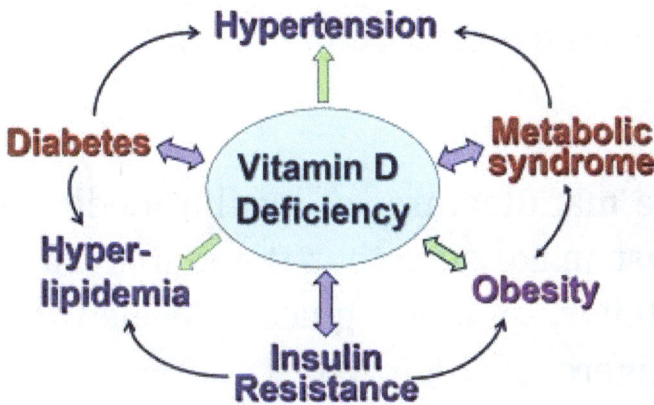

Insulin is not OK to use if exposed to very hot or cold weather. The three drug manufacturers of insulin in the United States say UNOPENED insulin is best stored inside the fridge [2° to 8°Celcius (36° to 46°Fahrenheit)].

UNOPENED insulin stored in the refrigerator is good until the expiration date printed on the insulin box. The expiration date will usually be 1 year from the date of purchase but you have to check the box to find out.

The manufacturer of insulin medication must make sure that the stuff is at full potency, or blood glucose levels can go dangerously high.

They must guarantee that their products will work as indicated if used within the expiration date and for not more than a month after the seal on the vial, cartridge, or pen is broken. This is, of course, assuming that the insulin has been stored properly and not exposed to extreme heat, freezing cold, or direct sunlight.

This does not mean that insulin suddenly goes bad at the stroke of midnight on the expiration date, or 28 days after being opened. Many people and clinicians with diabetes have used insulin beyond the expiration date, but there is no guarantee that the insulin remains at full strength.

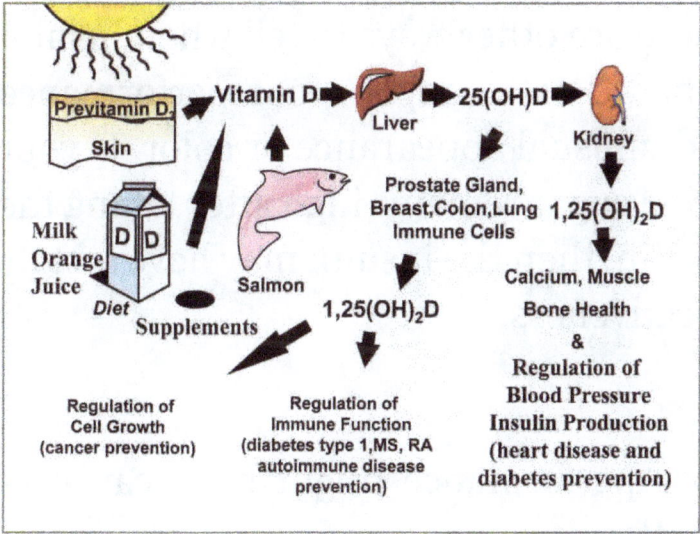

How know if the Insulin is Bad

The best way is to not use bottled insulin past the expiration date printed on the label. And no matter what the expiration date is, throw away a bottle one month after you open it. Write the date that you opened the bottle on the bottle's label.

There are other ways to tell when insulin is bad. For example, poor performance and unusual appearance or color. If your blood sugar remains high after taking the insulin, then the insulin may have lost its effectiveness.

Poor performance might be because of two things:

1. The insulin bottle was opened for more than 28 days.

2. There are lots of punctures, holes in the bottle's rubber stopper because you take small doses of insulin and you are now close to the end of the bottle.

If the insulin has an unusual appearance. For example, the insulin is cloudy when it is supposed to be clear, or the insulin has changed in color.

Your diet is also very important. The human body uses insulin to break down carbohydrates. Then a low carb-protein rich diet keeps your insulin dependency a more under control. If you are on a protein-rich diet, you should drink lots of water to help your blood from becoming too acidic. Also if it helps, try to drink a solution of sodium bicarbonate (baking soda). Baking soda will alkalize the body, which is the opposite of acidification.

Try to maintain your weight by eating many small meals during the day, try protein rich meals and as little carbs as possible. Avoid heavy-duty activities that might drain your body of energy. And always keep an eye on the symptoms of hyper/hypoglycemia by checking your blood sugar. Please see a doctor if you have symptoms like dizziness, fatigue, erratic heartbeat, confusion and even the loss of consciousness.

How To Make Insulin

Is it possible to make insulin for a long-term survival scenario? Yes, but it is not a very simple task. It is complicated and you will need access to some equipment.

These are some oral medication that can replace insulin by reducing the body's insulin resistance. Such medication often have a very long shelf life so we can easily store them. In this way, even the smallest quantities of insulin that the body might produce will help to lowering the blood sugar levels. The most important thing is to always try to help the body make its own insulin by providing it with the proper diet and also with a little help from some of the over-the-counter medication, like Metformin, NovoNorm, and Berberine. Buy the ones with the highest dosage available.

Berberine For Diabetes

A Natural Alternative to **Metformin**?

The current popular glucose-lowering drug treatment, Metformin comes with some potential serious side effects. However, there is a natural Metformin alternative that can help the body efficiently process sugar, thereby being safer than pharmaceutical interventions. It is known as Berberine.

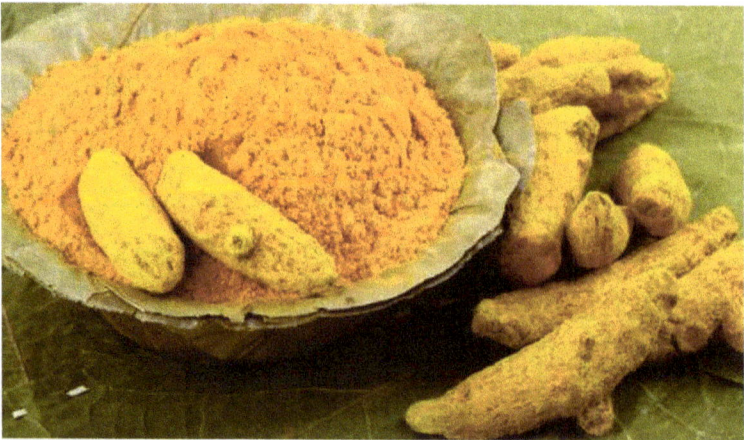

Berberine is a plant photochemical that is found in different plants, including goldenseal, European barberry, phellodendron, goldthread, Oregon grape, and tree turmeric.

Berberine possesses powerful anti-diabetic properties, as well as being anti-bacterial and immune system enhancing. As well as diabetes it can be used as a treatment for a number of other health problems including hyperlipidemia, heart disease, and cancer. It can regulate blood glucose, increase insulin sensitivity as well as metabolizing fats (burning fat). Berberine has been widely studied, with nearly 1000 studies published on it in the last 5 years alone. There is a body of evidence supporting it's efficacy in lowering blood-glucose and increasing insulin sensitivity for both humans and animals.

Mrs. Eva Saxl

I have read stories about Eva Saxl (1921-2002). She was a self-taught maker of insulin and an advocate for people with diabetes. Eva and her husband were born in Prague, Czechoslovakia. During World War II she and her husband, Victor Saxl, fled to Shanghai, China. In Shanghai Saxl was diagnosed with type 1 diabetes and followed by more bad luck. When the Japanese attacked Pearl Harbor in 1941, the Japanese occupation of China was tightened, and soon after that most all pharmacies in Shanghai were shut.

Eva had no legal access to insulin. It was possible to only buy insulin on the black market and by using only one-ounce gold bars for payment.

But that was never the safest option, because Eva's friend died from using the black market insulin.

Ultimately, Victor and Eva decided to get insulin in another way. They wanted to make it themselves. They used the book Beckman's Internal Medicine. The book described the methods that Dr. Frederick Banting and Charles Best first used to extract insulin from the pancreases of mammals, pigs, calves, and cows in 1921.

A kind Chinese chemist lent them a small laboratory. The laboratory was located in the basement of a municipal building. They attempted to extract insulin from pancreata of water buffaloes, and after much work, they were able to produce a brown-colored insulin.

The insulin was tested on rats starved for 24 hours. The rats were divided into two groups. One group was injected with the extracted mix, and the other with Eva's insulin.

Without equipment to test the rats' urine or blood, the best way Victor could test the potency of their insulin was to see if the rat's would experience the same kind of hypoglycaemic shock as the other rats. However, after testing the insulin on rats for more than a year, Eva was running out of her conventional insulin and so she cautiously tried it on herself, and it really worked.

In the Jewish neighborhood where they were living, many other people with type 1 diabetes were also in dire need of insulin. So very kind Eva gave her insulin to two boys in a nearby hospital who were in diabetic comas.

With many other very successful batches of homemade insulin, the Saxl's began production of insulin for all people with diabetes in their neighborhood.

In all, over 200 people, with thanks to Eva and her husband, survived between 1941 and 1945 and it was said that there were no fatalities reported as a result of tainted insulin.

Eva and her husband then left Shanghai after World War II and immigrated to the United States. Eva became the first vocal spokesperson for juvenile diabetes, and her husband Victor found work in the United Nations. When Victor Saxl died, Eva moved to live with her only living relative, her brother, in Santiago, Chile. There Eva also an advocate for people with diabetes. Eva Saxl died in 2002 in Santiago.

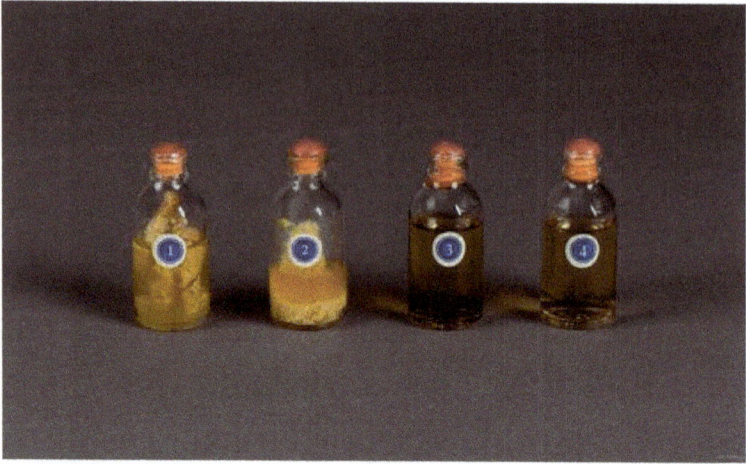

These vials of insulin come from an insulin sales kit made by Eli Lilly & Company in the 1940s (pictured below).

The numbers labeling the vials indicate a four-step progression as the insulin is manufactured into its final product.

Since the discovery of insulin in 1922 by a team of Canadian researchers, making insulin for the treatment of diabetes has always depended on living organisms.

Before the advent of biotechnology, the organisms used were the pigs and cows destined for our dinner plates— specifically, their pancreas glands, a waste product of the meatpacking industry.

More than two tons of pig parts were needed to extract just eight ounces of purified insulin. Lucky for us, both pork- and beef-derived insulin are nearly identical to human insulin and can be utilized by our bodies to convert the carbohydrates we eat into energy.

The crude process of extracting insulin from piles of animal glands may bother our sensibilities today, but also remember that diabetes used to be a death sentence; insulin dramatically restored life to children on the brink of starvation because of this disease.

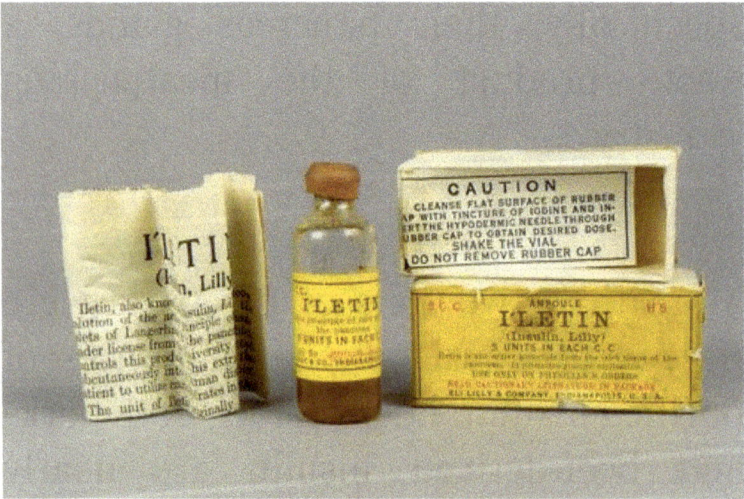

A bottle of 1920s Iletin (Lilly insulin), which is the finished product seen below being labeled and packaged.

Making Insulin At Home

To learn how to make insulin, try to read lectures about how the first insulin was created in the lab in 1922. The modern method of extracting insulin from genetically engineered bacteria or yeast will not be possible. Most people will not be able to get the equipment needed, and also the rich companies that make insulin will not give out samples of the bioengineered bacteria critters that create insulin from yeast. Therefore, our only option is to extract insulin from the pancreas of animals. Please do not harm them just for fun. Do this only if you have no other options. Please note that in order of preference, you can use pig, cow, sheep, goat, and then any other mammal that you can get. Fish also have a form of insulin, but not much, and not very potent in humans.

So to make insulin you will need to get some pancreatic organs of pigs or cows. You will also need some electric power in order to use a centrifuge, lab equipment, and also it would help a lot if you have great Chemistry knowledge.

It is highly unlikely that most people can manage to make insulin on their own, to put together all the chemicals and all the equipment in a disaster-scenario, but maybe you can do it.

Now let me explain to you the lecture from the 1920's, which was presented by the actual insulin inventors when they described how the insulin was created.

The 1920 Method to Make Insulin

The method of preparation is as follows First a summary of the preparation of the extracts as used in the first clinical cases:

To a small volume of 95%, ethyl alcohol freshly minced mammal's pancreas was added in equal amount. The mixture was then allowed to sit for some hours with occasional stirring and shaking. Then it was strained through a clean cheese cloth and the liquid part at once was filtered. The filtrate was then mixed (treated) with two volumes of 95 %, ethyl alcohol. By this the major part of the protein was removed, but the active important part remained in alcoholic solution. After allowing a few hours for the protein precipitation to be effected, the mixture was again filtered.

The filtrate concentrated to small bulk by distillation in vacuo at a low temperature (18° to 30°C, 64°F to 86°F).

The lipoid substances were then removed by twice extracting it with Sulphuric ether in a separating funnel, then the watery solution returned to the vacuum, where it was further concentrated until it was of a pasty consistency.

We added 80% ethyl alcohol, and the mixture was centrifuged again. After centrifuging, four distinct layers were manifested in the tube: The uppermost was perfectly clear and consisted of alcohol holding all the active principle in solution. Below this layer, in order, were a flocculent layer of protein, and a second clear watery layer saturated with salt, and then a lowermost layer consisting of crystals of salt.

The alcohol layer was then removed by means of a pipette and then was at once delivered into several volumes of 95%, alcohol, or better, of absolute alcohol.

We found that after this final treatment with alcohol of high grade, it caused the precipitation of the active principle along with adherent substances.

Some hours after this final precipitation, the precipitate was caught on a Buchner Funnel, dissolved in distilled water and then concentrated to the desired degree by use of the vacuum still. Finally, it was then passed through a Berkfeld filter, then sterility tests made and then the final product delivered to the clinic.

A more detailed summary:

The pig or cow pancreas is finely minced in a large grinder. The minced material parts is then treated with 5 c.c. of concentrated Sulphuric Acid, which is appropriately diluted, per pound of pancreas glands.

The mixture is then stirred for about 3 to 4 hours and then 95% alcohol is added until the concentration of alcohol is 60% to 70%.

Now two extractions of the glands are done. The solid gland material is partially removed by centrifuging the mixture, and the solution must be further clarified by filtering through paper.

Next the filtrate is practically neutralized with Sodium Hydroxide.

The clear filtrate is concentrated in vacuo to about 1/15 of its original volume. The concentrate is then heated to about 50 degrees Centigrade, which results in the separation of lipoid and the other materials, are removed by filtration.

Ammonium sulphate (37 grams. per 100 c.c.) is then added to the concentrate. A protein material which contain all the Insulin floats to the top of the liquid.

The precipitate is then skimmed off and dissolved in hot acid alcohol. And when the precipitate has completely dissolved, add 10 volumes of warm alcohol.

The solution is then neutralized with sodium hydroxide (NaOH) and cooled to room temperature, and kept in a refrigerator at 5 C (41 F) for two days.

At the end of two days, the dark colored supernatant alcohol is decanted off. The alcohol contains practically no potency.

The precipitate is then dried in vacuo to remove all trace of the alcohol.

Next it is dissolved in acid water, in which it is readily soluble. The solution is then made alkaline with sodium hydroxide (NaOH) to PH 7.3 to 7.5. At this alkalinity a dark colored precipitate will settle out, and then it is immediately centrifuged off.

This precipitate is then washed once or twice with alkaline water of PH 9.0, and the washings are then added to the main liquid.

It is **<u>extremely</u>** important that this process is carried out very quickly because Insulin is destroyed in alkaline solution. The acidity is adjusted to PH 5.0 and a white precipitate readily settles out.

Tricresol is then added to a concentration of 0.3% in order to assist in the isoelectric precipitation and to act as a preservative.

After standing for about one week in an ice chest, the supernatant liquid is then decanted off and the resultant liquid is removed by centrifuging. The precipitate is then dissolved in a small quantity of acid water.

Now a second isoelectric precipitation is carried out by adjusting the acidity to a PH of approximately 5.0.

Next after standing for over a night the resultant precipitate is then removed by centrifuging.

The precipitate, which will contain the active principle in a comparatively pure form, is then dissolved in acid water and the hydrogen ion concentration adjusted to PH 2.5.

The material is then carefully tested to determine the potency, then it is diluted to the desired strength of 10, 20, 40 or 80 units per c.c.

Tricresol is then added to get and secure a concentration of 0.1 percent.

Sufficient sodium chloride is then added to make the solution isotonic.

Finally, pass the solution which contains the Insulin through a Mandler filter.

After passing the solution through the filter, the Insulin is retested carefully to determine its potency.

There is practically no loss in berkefeld filtering.

The tested Insulin can then be poured into sterile glass vials with aseptic precautions.

The sterility of the final Insulin product must be thoroughly tested by approved methods.

A last note on insulin thermo stability

Some researcher state that commercial Insulin is generally more stable and hearty than the label suggests (i.e. 30 days).

Doctors Without Borders commissioned a study to examine the loss of potency. Though heat will denature insulin it has to be pretty intense for long periods of time.

Sunlight and shaking will also destroy potency. However in most cases a person can get months of potency even if it is kept outside of a fridge.

However, what will quickly destroy the insulin though is going the other way – freezing. So be careful not to store directly on ice packs.

Basic Principles of Ventilator Design

A ventilator is a machine that provides mechanical ventilation by moving breathable air into and out of the lungs, to deliver breaths to a patient who is physically unable to breathe, or breathing insufficiently.

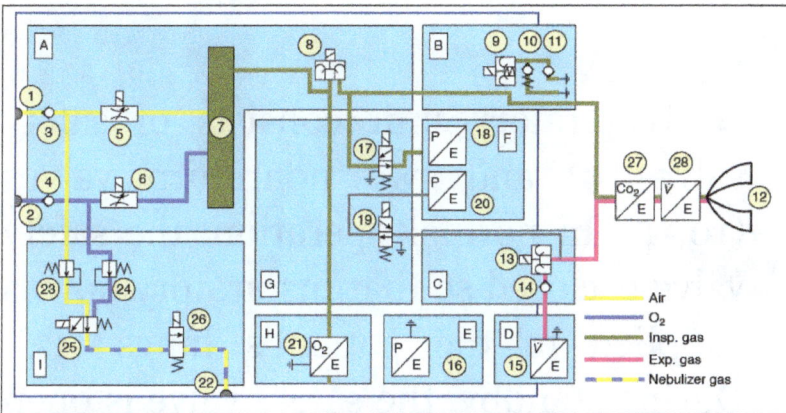

1 Air gas inlet	16 Barometric pressure sensor
2 O_2 gas inlet	17 Calibration valve for inspiratory pressure sensor
3 Air nonreturn valve	18 Inspiratory pressure sensor
4 O_2 nonreturn valve	19 Calibration valve for expiratory pressure sensor
5 Air metering valve	20 Expiratory pressure sensor
6 O_2 metering valve	21 O_2 sensor
7 Tank	22 Nebulizer outlet
8 Mixed gas metering valve	23 Air pressure regulator
9 Safety valve	24 O_2 pressure regulator
10 Emergency expiratory valve	25 Nebulizer mixer valve
11 Emergency breathing valve	26 Nebulizer changeover valve
12 Patient's lungs	27 CO_2 sensor
13 Expiratory valve	28 Neonatal flow sensor (depending on the patient category)
14 Nonreturn valve	
15 Expiratory flow sensor	

A. Gas-mixture and gas-metering assembly. Gas from the supply lines enters the ventilator via the gas-inlet connections for oxygen and air (1,2). Two nonreturn valves (3,4) prevent one gas from returning to the supply line of the other gas. Mixing takes place in the tank (7) and is controlled by two valves (5,6). Inspiratory flow is controlled by a third valve (8).

B. Inspiratory unit consists of safety valve (9) and two nonreturn valves (10,11). In normal operation, the safety valve is closed so that inspiratory flow is supplied to the patient's lungs (12). During standby, the safety valve is open and enables spontaneous inspiration by the emergency breathing valve (11). The emergency expiratory valve (10) provides a second channel for expiration when the expiratory valve (13) is blocked.

C. Expiratory unit consists of the expiratory valve (13) and a non-return valve (14). The expiratory valve is a proportional valve and is used to adjust the pressure in the patient circuit. In conjunction with the spring-loaded valve of the emergency air outlet (10), the nonreturn valve (14) prevents pendulum breathing during spontaneous breathing.

D. Expiratory flow sensor.

E. Barometric pressure sensor. Conversion of mass flow to volume, body temperature and pressure saturated (BTPS) requires knowledge of ambient pressure.

F. Pressure measurement assembly. Pressure in the patient circuit is measured with two independent pressure sensors (18,20).

G. Calibration assembly. The pressure sensors are regularly zero calibrated by connection to ambient pressure via the two calibration valves (17,19).

H. Oxygen sensor.

I. Medication nebulizer assembly.

Inputs

Mechanical ventilators are typically powered by electricity or compressed gas. Electricity, either from wall outlets (e.g., 100 to 240 volts AC, at 50/60 Hz) or from batteries (e.g., 10 to 30 volts DC), is used to run compressors of various types. These sources provide compressed air for motive power as well as air for breathing. Alternatively, the power to expand the lungs is supplied by compressed gas from tanks, or from wall outlets in the hospital (e.g., 30 to 80 pounds per square inch [psi]). Some transport and emergency ventilators use compressed gas to power both lung inflation and the control circuitry. For these ventilators, knowledge of gas consumption is critical when using cylinders of compressed gas.

The ventilator is generally connected to separate sources of compressed air and compressed oxygen. In the United States, hospital wall outlets supply air and oxygen at 50 psi, although most ventilators have internal regulators to reduce this pressure to a lower level (e.g., 20 psi). This permits the delivery of a range of oxygen concentrations to support the needs of sick patients. Because compressed gas has all moisture removed, the gas delivered to the patient must be warmed and humidified so as to avoid drying out the lung tissue.

Conversion and Control

The input power of a ventilator must be converted to a predefined output of pressure and flow. There are several key systems required for this process.

If the only power input is electrical, the ventilator must use a compressor or blower to generate the required pressure and flow. A compressor is a machine for moving a relatively low flow of gas to a storage container at a higher level of pressure (e.g., 20 psi). A blower is a machine for generating relatively larger flows of gas as the direct ventilator output with a relatively moderate increase of pressure (e.g., 2 psi). Compressors are generally found on intensive care ventilators whereas blowers are used on home-care and transport ventilators. Compressors are typically larger and consume more electrical power than blowers, hence the use of the latter on small, portable devices.

Flow-Control Valves

To control the flow of gas from a compressor, ventilator engineers use a variety of flow-control valves, from very simple to very complex. The simplest valve is just a fixed orifice flow resistor that permits setting a constant flow to the external tubing that conducts the gas to the patient, called the patient circuit. Such devices are used in small transport ventilators and automatic resuscitators.

The advent of inexpensive microprocessors in the late 1970s led to development of digital control of flow valves that allow a great deal of flexibility in shaping the ventilator's output pressure, volume, and flow waveforms (Fig 3-4).

Such valves are used in most of the current generation of intensive care ventilators.

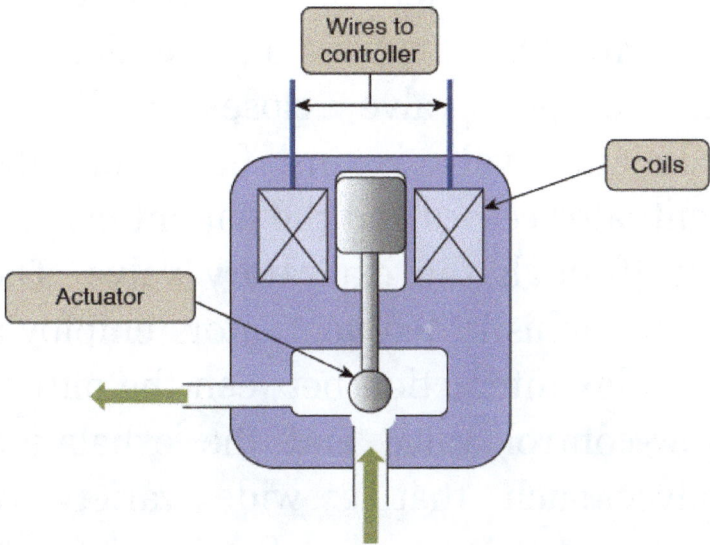

3-4: Schematic of an output flow-control valve.

Directing flow from the source gas into the patient requires the coordination of the output flow-control valve and an expiratory valve or "exhalation manifold" (Fig. 3-5).

In the simplest case, when inspiration is triggered on, the output control valve opens, the expiratory valve closes, and the only path left for gas is into the patient. When inspiration is cycled off, the output valve closes and the exhalation valve opens, flow from the ventilator ceases and the patient exhales out through the expiratory valve. The most sophisticated ventilators employ a complex interaction between the output flow-control valve and the exhalation valve, such that a wide variety of pressure, volume, and flow waveforms may be generated to synchronize the ventilator output with patient effort as much as possible.

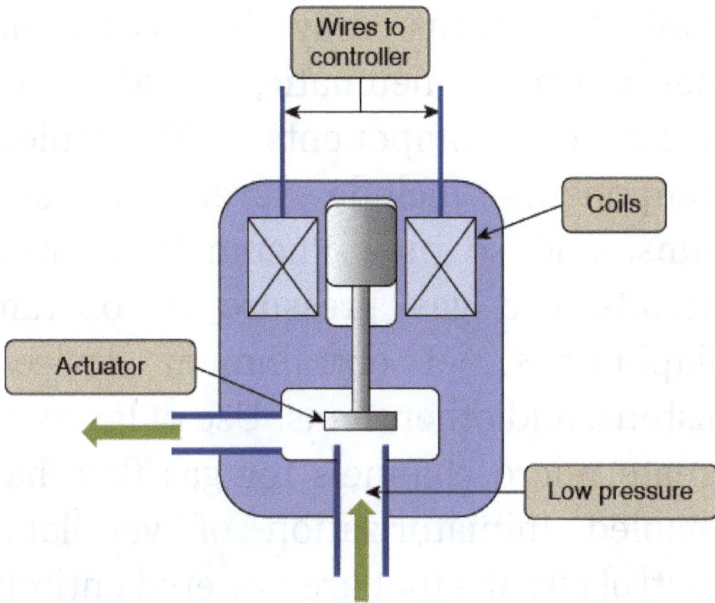

3.5: Schematic of an exhalation valve.

Control Systems

In the simplest terms, the control system of a ventilator is comprised of components that generate the signals that operate the output valve and the exhalation manifold to obtain the desired output waveforms and modes of ventilation.

Control systems may be based on mechanical, pneumatic, fluidic, or electronic components. Mechanical components include levers, pulleys, cams, and so on.3 Pneumatic control circuits use gas pressure to operate diaphragms, jet entrainment devices, pistons, and other items. Use of lasers to create micro channels for gas flow has enabled miniaturization of ventilator control circuits that are powered entirely by gas pressure to create small, but sophisticated, ventilators for transport. Fluidic circuits are analogs of electronic logic circuits. Just as an electronic logic circuit uses electricity, the fluidic circuit uses a very small gas flows to generate signals that operate switches and timing components. Both pneumatic and fluidic control systems are immune to failure from electromagnetic interference, such as around magnetic resonance imaging equipment.

Examples of simple pneumatic and fluidic ventilator control circuits have been illustrated elsewhere. By far, the majority of ventilators use electronic control circuits with microprocessors to manage the complex monitoring (e.g., from pressure and flow sensors) and control (valves) functions of modern ventilators used in almost every health care environment.

What makes one ventilator so different from another has as much to do with the control system software as it does with the hardware. The control software determines how the ventilator interacts with the patient; that is, the modes available. Thus, a discussion about control systems is essentially a discussion about mode capabilities and classifications.

Outputs

Just as the study of cardiology involves the use of electrocardiograms and blood pressure waveforms, the study of mechanical ventilation requires an understanding of output waveforms. The waveforms of interest are the pressure, volume, and flow.

Position Virus/Lung Patients on their Stomach can save their Life

If you place the sickest Lung / Virus patients on their stomachs, called prone positioning, helps **increase the amount of oxygen** that's getting to their lungs.

Once you see it work, you will want to do it more, and you see it work almost immediately. You are opening up parts of the lung.

Patients with Lung / Virus illness often die of ARDS, or acute respiratory distress syndrome. The same syndrome also kills patients who have influenza, pneumonia and other diseases.

The New England Journal of Medicine showed that patients with ARDS who were on ventilators had a lower chance of dying if they were placed on their stomachs in the hospital.

When the patients are placed on their stomach, their oxygen saturation rate, a measure of oxygen in the blood, will go from 85% to 98%, a huge jump.

The ventilated patients typically stay on their stomachs for about 16 hours a day, going on their backs for the rest of the time so doctors have better access to their front side and can more easily give them the treatments they need.

Critical care specialists say being on the belly seems help because it allows oxygen to more easily get to the lungs. While on the back, the weight of the body in effect squishes some sections of the lungs.

By putting them on their stomachs, you are opening up parts of the lung that weren't open before.

Choosing belly or back

There is a downside to placing ventilated Lung / Virus patients on their stomachs. Ventilated patients require more sedation when they are on their stomachs, which could mean a longer stay in the ICU. About a third of the patients on ventilators get placed on their stomachs, usually the ones who are sickest and have the most to gain from being in that position.

It might be uncomfortable for a non-sedated patient to spend 16 hours on their stomachs, so try to get them to spend at least four hours on the stomachs, split into two sessions.

How long they stay in that position really varies from person to person, whether they're comfortable falling asleep in that position, or if they get bored and want to turn over to their backs.

A French study looked only at patients who were on ventilators, so it's not entirely clear what effecting the stomach position has for patients who are not as severely ill.